Comprehensive Primer on EUS-Guided Tissue Acquisition

Editors

SHYAM VARADARAJULU
ROBERT H. HAWES

GASTROINTESTINAL ENDOSCOPY CLINICS OF NORTH AMERICA

www.giendo.theclinics.com

Consulting Editor
CHARLES J. LIGHTDALE

January 2014 • Volume 24 • Number 1

ELSEVIER

1600 John F. Kennedy Boulevard ● Suite 1800 ● Philadelphia, Pennsylvania, 19103-2899

http://www.theclinics.com

GASTROINTESTINAL ENDOSCOPY CLINICS OF NORTH AMERICA Volume 24, Number 1
January 2014 ISSN 1052-5157, ISBN-13: 978-0-323-26390-0

Editor: Kerry Holland
Developmental Editor: Donald Mumford

Gastrointestinal Endoscopy Clinics of North America (ISSN 1052-5157) is published quarterly by Elsevier Inc., 360 Park Avenue South, New York, NY 10010-1710. Months of issue are January, April, July, and October. Business and Editorial Offices: 1600 John F. Kennedy Blvd., Suite 1800, Philadelphia, PA, 19103-2899. Periodicals postage paid at New York, NY and additional mailing offices. Subscription prices are $335.00 per year for US individuals, $486.00 per year for US institutions, $175.00 per year for US students and residents, $370.00 per year for Canadian individuals, $576.00 per year for Canadian institutions, $465.00 per year for international individuals, $576.00 per year for international institutions, and $245.00 per year for Canadian and foreign students/residents. To receive student/resident rate, orders must be accompanied by name of affiliated institution, date of term, and the signature of program/residency coordinator on institution letterhead. Orders will be billed at individual rate until proof of status is received. Foreign air speed delivery is included in all Clinics subscription prices. All prices are subject to change without notice. **POSTMASTER:** Send address change to Gastrointestinal Endoscopy Clinics of North America, Elsevier Health Sciences Division, Subscription Customer Service, 3251 Riverport Lane, Maryland Heights, MO 63043. **Customer Service: 1-800-654-2452 (US). From outside the United States, call 1-314-447-8871. Fax: 1-314-447-8029. E-mail: JournalsCustomerService-usa@elsevier.com (for print support) or JournalsOnlineSupport-usa@elsevier.com (for online support).**

Reprints. For copies of 100 or more, of articles in this publication, please contact the Commercial Reprints Department, Elsevier Inc., 360 Park Avenue South, New York, NY 10010-1710. Tel. 212-633-3874; Fax: 212-633-3820; E-mail: reprints@elsevier.com.

Gastrointestinal Endoscopy Clinics of North America is covered in Excerpta Medica, MEDLINE/PubMed (Index Medicus), and MEDLINE/MEDLARS.

Printed and bound by CPI Group (UK) Ltd, Croydon, CR0 4YY

Transferred to digital print 2012

Contributors

CONSULTING EDITOR

CHARLES J. LIGHTDALE, MD
Professor, Department of Medicine, Columbia University Medical Center, New York, New York

EDITORS

SHYAM VARADARAJULU, MD
Medical Director of Endoscopy, Center for Interventional Endoscopy, Florida Hospital, Orlando, Florida

ROBERT H. HAWES, MD
Medical Director, Institute For Minimally Invasive Therapy, Florida Hospital, Orlando, Florida

AUTHORS

MOHAMMAD AL-HADDAD, MD, MSC, FASGE
Associate Professor of Medicine, Division of Gastroenterology and Hepatology, Indiana University School of Medicine, Indianapolis, Indiana

J. PABLO ARNOLETTI, MD
Professor of Surgery, Florida State University, Professor of Surgery, University of Central Florida, Florida Hospital Orlando, Orlando, Florida

SEBASTIAN G. DE LA FUENTE, MD
Assistant Professor of Surgery, Florida State University, and Assistant Professor of Surgery, University of Central Florida, Florida Hospital Orlando, Orlando, Florida

PIERRE H. DEPREZ, MD, PhD
Department of Hepato-Gastroenterology, Cliniques Universitaires Saint-Luc, Université Catholique de Louvain, Brussels, Belgium

LARISSA L. FUJII, MD
Division of Gastroenterology and Hepatology, Mayo Clinic, Rochester, Minnesota

ROBERT H. HAWES, MD
Medical Director, Institute For Minimally Invasive Therapy, Florida Hospital, Orlando, Florida

SHANTEL HÉBERT-MAGEE, MD
Assistant Professor, Department of Pathology, University of Alabama at Birmingham, Birmingham, Alabama

DARSHANA JHALA, MD, BMus
Associate Professor of Pathology, Department of Pathology and Laboratory Medicine, Director of Anatomic Pathology, Philadelphia Veterans Affairs Medical Center, University of Pennsylvania, Philadelphia, Pennsylvania

NIRAG JHALA, MD, MIAC
Professor of Pathology and Laboratory Medicine, Director of Cytopathology, Department of Pathology and Laboratory Medicine, University of Pennsylvania, Philadelphia, Pennsylvania

ZEID KARADSHEH, MD
Department of Internal Medicine, Brockton Hospital, Brockton, Massachusetts

ALBERTO LARGHI, MD, PhD
Director of the Endoscopic Ultrasound Program, Digestive Endoscopy Unit, Catholic University, Rome, Italy

MICHAEL J. LEVY, MD
Division of Gastroenterology and Hepatology, Mayo Clinic, Rochester, Minnesota

NIKOLA PANIC, MD
Digestive Endoscopy Unit, Catholic University, Rome, Italy; Department of Medicine, University of Belgrade, Belgrade, Serbia

SARTO C. PAQUIN, MD, FRCPC
Centre hospitalier de l'Université de Montréal, Montréal, Québec, Canada

ADRIAN SĂFTOIU, MD, PhD, MSc, FASGE
Visiting Clinical Professor, Department of Endoscopy, Gastrointestinal Unit, Copenhagen University Hospital, Herlev, Denmark; Professor, Department of Gastroenterology, Research Center of Gastroenterology and Hepatology, Craiova, Romania

ANAND V. SAHAI, MD, MSc (EPID), FRCPC
Centre hospitalier de l'Université de Montréal, Montréal, Québec, Canada

ANDRADA SEICEAN, MD, PhD, FASGE
Associate Professor of Gastroenterology, Department of Gastroenterology, Regional Institute of Gastroenterology and Hepatology, University of Medicine and Pharmacy, Cluj-Napoca, Romania

SHYAM VARADARAJULU, MD
Medical Director of Endoscopy, Center for Interventional Endoscopy, Florida Hospital, Orlando, Florida

PETER VILMANN, MD, DSc, FASGE
Professor of Endoscopy, Department of Endoscopy, Gastrointestinal Unit, Copenhagen University Hospital, Herlev, Denmark

Contents

The diagnostic performance of endoscopic ultrasound-guided fine-needle aspiration is strongly dependent on the availability of an onsite cytopathologist. The diagnosis of some rare tumors may require ancillary testing for which a histologic core biopsy is required. There is increasing interest in evaluating core tissue for molecular markers that may serve as prognostic predictors and targets for focused chemotherapy in patients with cancer. If core tissue can be procured efficiently and reliably at endoscopic ultrasound, this will eliminate the need for an onsite cytopathologist, accurately diagnose tumors that are occasionally missed by fine-needle aspiration cytology, and enable the assessment for molecular markers.

There are 2 main reasons why oncologists may require additional tissue and a histologic section in addition to cytopathology from fine-needle aspiration (FNA) specimens: improved diagnostic accuracy and molecular characterization of tumors. Rather than mutually exclusive diagnostic procedures, endoscopic ultrasound (EUS)-FNA and EUS- core needle biopsy must be viewed as supplementary techniques and both approaches should be incorporated as essential tools in the current endoscopic armamentarium.

This article identifies key fundamentals of tissue acquisition, sample preparation, and staining. It defines the understanding of different aspects of sample preparations, such as types of smear-preparation techniques, touch preparations, types of fixative, and newer technologies such as liquid-based preparations.

Endoscopic ultrasound-guided fine-needle aspiration (EUS-FNA) has become well established as a minimally invasive technique in diagnosing and staging various gastrointestinal, pancreaticobiliary, and retroperitoneal malignancies. The diagnostic accuracy of this procedure is significantly enhanced by the presence of on-site cytopathology. However, in many EUS centers, cytopathology is not readily available for on-site evaluation. This article is intended to assist the independent endosonographer in the assessment of diagnostic sufficiency and in specimen handling.

 Videos of the fanning technique and the uncinate process accompany this article

Endoscopic ultrasound-guided fine-needle aspiration (EUS-FNA) is increasingly used as a diagnostic and therapeutic tool for pancreatic and other gastrointestinal disorders. Several factors affect the outcome of EUS-FNA, one of which is needle size. The decision to use a specific needle depends on factors including location, consistency, and type of the lesion; presence of onsite cytopathologist; and need for additional tissue procurement for histology. This review provides a balanced perspective on the use of different needle sizes available, highlighting the differences among them and potential niche applications of each to maximize diagnostic yield of EUS-FNA.

This article addresses the technique of endoscopic ultrasound-guided fine-needle aspiration of solid lesions to obtain cytologic specimens. The technique can be broken down into a sequence of steps. The ultimate goal is to maximize the likelihood of obtaining adequate tissue for diagnostic purposes. This requires a technique that ensures that the needle can be moved inside the lesion, under ultrasound guidance, as widely as possible, as easily as possible, and safely. The other variables such as suction, needle type, and stylet use are of secondary importance.

Although endoscopic ultrasound-guided fine-needle aspiration (EUS-FNA) is the method of choice to obtain samples to reach definitive diagnosis of lesions of the gastrointestinal tract and of adjacent organs, it cannot fully characterize certain neoplasms. The lack of cytology expertise has hindered the dissemination of EUS, limiting its widespread use. Obtaining a tissue specimen through EUS fine-needle biopsy (EUS-FNB) may overcome the limitations of EUS-FNA. EUS-FNB is expected to move the practice of EUS from cytology to histology, expanding the use of EUS and facilitating targeted therapies and monitoring of treatment response in a more biologically driven manner.

The diagnostic yield of EUS-FNA depends on several factors, such as the experience of the endosonographer, the characteristics of the lesion, the clinical status of the patient, the size and type of needles, the methods of specimen preparation, as well as cytopathologist expertise. The endosonographic technique can be improved when several tips and tricks useful to overcome challenges of FNA are known. Technical challenges of FNA are related to the characteristics of the lesion and its surroundings, sonographic imaging, and limitations related to the needle. Several tips and tricks necessary to overcome them are presented in this review.

Although endoscopic ultrasound (EUS) fine-needle aspiration (FNA) is a safe and accurate procedure, the diagnostic yield varies. Factors contributing to the diagnostic accuracy of EUS FNA include endosonographer and cytopathologist experience, EUS image recognition, accurate FNA targeting of the lesion, proper specimen collection and handling, use of ancillary techniques, and accurate cytologic interpretation. Errors in performance or judgment made before, during, or after the procedure may affect the results of the EUS FNA. The authors discuss the potential pitfalls of EUS FNA and methods to avoid their occurrence to optimize the diagnostic yield, efficiency, and safety of the procedure.

Endoscopic ultrasound fine-needle aspiration is considered the technique of choice for acquisition of tissue in and around the digestive tract. The emergence of selective, targeted therapies, directed toward a particular molecular characteristic of an individual patient's tumor is driving the need for biomarker identification and testing in several cancer types. The technique needs improvement to provide more material, in fewer passes, with more flexible, sharp, and clearly echovisible needles, and with a similar safety. Another trend is the avoidance of tissue acquisition, or a more targeted puncture with the help of ancillary techniques, such as optical biopsies with needle-based confocal laser endomicroscopy, contrast-enhanced ultrasonography, and elastography.

GASTROINTESTINAL ENDOSCOPY CLINICS OF NORTH AMERICA

Foreword

New Methods to Obtain Better Tissue Samples with EUS-guided FNA

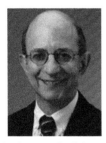

Charles J. Lightdale, MD
Consulting Editor

Endoscopic ultrasound (EUS) started out as primarily an imaging technique, but it soon became clear that EUS-guided fine-needle aspiration (FNA) for tissue acquisition would become a dominant function. Walking past an endoscopy room, one might hear phrases like "dart-throw" or "ice-pick" as we tried to teach GI Fellows how to use various EUS needles more notable for their similarities than their differences.

There was some early hope that computer analysis of ultrasound signals might reveal "signatures" correlating with specific diagnoses. Although some progress has been made, that goal remains elusive. The successful alternative was EUS-guided FNA to obtain cytologic and histologic specimens from imaged abnormalities. The development of electronic linear ultrasound endoscopes, with the ultrasound beam parallel to the instrument channel, allowed EUS-guided FNA to be carried out with great precision. Linear EUS systems and scopes improved rapidly and have been widely adopted by interventional endoscopists with a focus on subepithelial wall lesions, lymph nodes, and especially the pancreas.

Interestingly, it is only in recent years that major improvements have been made to the needles used for EUS-guided FNA. In addition, there has been progress in the development of new techniques for better tissue acquisition in different circumstances. There is some disagreement among specialists on the choice of needles and methods. However, no one disagrees that obtaining adequate tissue to guide new individualized therapies in gastroenterology, surgery, and oncology has become of critical importance.

The Guest Editors for this issue of the *Gastrointestinal Endoscopy Clinics of North America* on "EUS-guided Tissue Acquisition" are Robert Hawes, a pioneer and world leader in the field of EUS, and his colleague, Shyam Varadarajulu, representing the next generation of endosonographer-interventionalists. They have assembled a group of

Gastrointest Endoscopy Clin N Am 24 (2014) ix–x
http://dx.doi.org/10.1016/j.giec.2013.08.012
1052-5157/14/$ – see front matter © 2014 Elsevier Inc. All rights reserved.

giendo.theclinics.com

experts who share their passion to obtain the best possible results from EUS-guided FNA, and they have compiled a volume that covers all the relevant topics and controversies.

The choices in carrying out EUS-guided FNA have become rather complex. There are a variety of needle designs now available that offer different advantages and possibilities. Hitting the target with the needle is obviously central to success, but only the first step in maximizing the likelihood of getting a sufficient specimen for an accurate diagnosis. Everything that you need to know to obtain an optimal sample is in this state-of-the-art volume. If you are performing or learning EUS-guided FNA, this issue of the *Gastrointestinal Endoscopy Clinics of North America* is a "don't miss."

Charles J. Lightdale, MD
Department of Medicine
Columbia University Medical Center
161 Fort Washington Avenue, Room 812
New York, NY 10032, USA

E-mail address:
CJL18@columbia.edu

Preface: EUS-Guided Tissue Acquisition

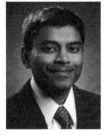 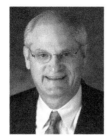

Shyam Varadarajulu, MD   Robert H. Hawes, MD
Editors

There has been a significant shift in the practice of EUS-guided tissue acquisition since the technique was first reported 21 years ago. The FNA needles are now available in different sizes, design, and flexibility. Depending on clinical need, both cytological aspirate and/or a histological core tissue can be procured with relative ease. Various techniques of tissue sampling have been described and validated in algorithms and clinical trials. These developments have enabled the establishment of a specific tissue diagnosis in a majority of patients, thereby enabling surgeons and oncologists to deliver "planned" treatment with optimal clinical outcomes. In addition to establishing cytologic or histologic diagnosis, we are now able to diagnose lymphomatous and other rare diseases as well as assess tumors for molecular markers to enable tailored chemotherapy regimens. However, despite these advances, certain limitations such as the dependence on an onsite cytopathologist for achieving high diagnostic accuracy, technical difficulty in accessing small pancreatic lesions in the uncinate process, inability to reliably procure core tissue, and controversies on the best technique to collect and process specimens still persist.

In this supplement of the *Gastrointestinal Endoscopy Clinics of North America* we have attempted to provide a comprehensive review of the existing practices in EUS-guided tissue acquisition and shed light on some of the controversies listed above. We hope this will serve as a valuable reference to enable you to improve your EUS service for the benefit of your patients. We are very grateful to the authors who have selflessly contributed to this issue to make our discipline better for tomorrow.

Shyam Varadarajulu, MD
Center for Interventional Endoscopy
Florida Hospital
601 East Rollins Street
Orlando, FL 32803, USA

Gastrointest Endoscopy Clin N Am 24 (2014) xi–xii
http://dx.doi.org/10.1016/j.giec.2013.08.011
1052-5157/14/$ – see front matter © 2014 Elsevier Inc. All rights reserved.

giendo.theclinics.com

Robert H. Hawes, MD
Institute for Minimally Invasive Therapy
Florida Hospital
601 East Rollins Street
Orlando, FL 32803, USA

E-mail addresses:
svaradarajulu@yahoo.com (S. Varadarajulu)
robert.hawesmd@gmail.com (R.H. Hawes)

The Changing Paradigm in EUS-Guided Tissue Acquisition

Shyam Varadarajulu, MD[a],*, Robert H. Hawes, MD[b]

KEYWORDS

- Endoscopic ultrasound • Fine-needle aspiration • Fine-needle biopsy • Core biopsy
- Tissue acquisition

KEY POINTS

- Endoscopic ultrasound-guided fine-needle aspiration (EUS-FNA) is an accurate technique for establishing tissue diagnosis in patients with tumors or lesions in or adjacent to the gastrointestinal tract.
- The diagnostic performance of EUS-FNA is strongly dependent on the availability of an onsite cytopathologist.
- The diagnosis of some rare tumors may require ancillary testing for which a histologic core biopsy is required.
- Within oncology, there has been increasing interest in evaluating core tissue for molecular markers that may serve as prognostic predictors and targets for focused chemotherapy in patients with cancer.

The impact of endoscopic ultrasound-guided fine-needle aspiration (EUS-FNA) on the practice of pancreatic pathology is considered a disruptive innovation.[1] EUS-FNA rightly fits the description of a disruptive technology: "technically straight forward, consisting of off-the-shelf components put together in a way that is often simpler than prior approaches."[2] EUS-FNA consists of three technologies, each of which is disruptive in its own way: fiberoptic endoscopy was disruptive to rigid endoscopy, ultrasound to radiograph, and cytology to histology.[1] A recent study analyzed the pattern of pancreatic pathology examinations during a 20-year period in a tertiary referral center with relationship to implementation of a EUS-FNA program.[1] The sensitivity and specificity for cancer diagnosis improved from 55% and 78% to 88% and 96%, respectively, after implementation of the EUS-FNA program. Unsatisfactory (7% vs 1%), atypical (16% vs 4%), and suspicious (16% vs 3%) diagnosis were

Disclosures: The authors are consultants for Boston Scientific Corporation and Olympus Medical Systems Corporation.
[a] Center for Interventional Endoscopy, Florida Hospital, 601 East Rollins Street, Orlando, FL 32803, USA; [b] Institute for Minimally Invasive Therapy, Florida Hospital, 601 East Rollins Street, Orlando, FL 32803, USA
* Corresponding author.
E-mail address: svaradarajulu@yahoo.com

significantly reduced. After implementation of the EUS-FNA program, whereas the average percentage of annual cases managed by cytology alone increased from 19% to 51%, the percentage managed by histology alone declined from 56% to 23%. Consequently, non–EUS-guided FNA cytology decreased from 36% to 1% and needle biopsies from 29% to 9%. Because EUS-FNA brought about a much-needed improvement in diagnostic accuracy, it resulted in the displacement of histologic diagnosis in management of pancreatic diseases. This is evident from a recent study conducted by these authors that examined the 5-year trend (2006–2010) in tissue acquisition in pancreatic diseases in the United States using the Medicare database: The use of EUS-FNA increased by 69.3%, surgical biopsy declined by 41.7%, and the use of percutaneous biopsy has remained stable.[3]

Although EUS-FNA can be regarded as a disruptive innovation, it is important for endosonographers to recognize the imperfections of EUS and make constant refinements and incremental improvements to existing techniques, technologies, and practice patterns. This self-evaluation is important because it enables one to see "what is next." This might occasionally result in technological development that is offered in excess of what the consumer (endosonographers) demands or needs. Herein, the consumer weighs-in to differentiate between a sustaining "valued-based" technology and just "another" technology. Although biased investigators and industry-driven studies may make this distinction difficult, fortunately in medicine only those technologies that impact patient care in a meaningful manner eventually withstand the test of time.

LIMITATIONS OF EUS-GUIDED FNA CYTOLOGY

There are three limitations to EUS-guided FNA that if overcome can propel the technology even further: (1) the availability of onsite cytopathology support, (2) the occasional dependence on histology to establish a diagnosis that is otherwise not possible with FNA cytology, and (3) the ability to reliably assess the tissue sample for molecular markers so that patients can be risk stratified and treated with tailored chemotherapeutic agents.

On-site Cytopathology Support

All studies have shown that the presence of an onsite cytopathologist improves the diagnostic yield, decreases the number of inadequate or unsatisfactory samples, and limits the number of FNA passes required to establish a diagnosis.[4–7] In addition, two recent meta-analyses on EUS-FNA of pancreatic masses reached the same conclusions: the presence of an onsite cytopathologist was associated with a diagnostic sensitivity of 88% to 95% compared with 80% or less in the absence of a cytopathologist.[8,9]

For institutions limited by resources, this challenge can be mitigated by adapting a combination of measures. (1) If the endosonographers have basic training in cytopathology to assess for onsite diagnostic adequacy, appropriate samples can be collected and sent for off-site assessment by a cytopathologist. In a recent study of 138 patients who underwent EUS-FNA of solid pancreatic mass lesions, two endosonographers underwent proctoring in cytopathology and found that by assessing for onsite diagnostic adequacy themselves, the rates of diagnostic accuracy improved by 22% and inconclusive diagnosis declined by 18%.[10] (2) If adequate FNA passes can be performed to provide an adequate cell block, a reliable diagnosis can be achieved in most patients. In a prospective study of 91 patients with pancreatic masses who underwent EUS-FNA using a 22-G or 25-G needle, two passes were made for cell block analysis.[11] The specimens were immediately fixed in formalin and processed later by the cell block method. By adapting this technique, adequate tissue was procured in 88 (97%) of 91 patients. Of these 88 patients, the accuracy of the cell block method for diagnosing carcinoma was 99% and for neuroendocrine tumor was 100%. The caveat with this method is that, in patients with large tumors, the aspirate may contain nonviable necrotic material and a cell block may still be nondiagnostic. (3) The need for an onsite cytopathologist can be obviated if reliable core tissue can be procured for histologic assessment. Currently, none of the specially designed biopsy needles or a 19-G needle can guarantee reliable histologic core tissue procurement or demonstrate a diagnostic accuracy of greater than 95%.[12–15]

For centers that do not have access to onsite cytopathology support, a combination of all three measures must be adopted to achieve a diagnostic accuracy of greater than 95%. The endosonographer after (self) assessing for diagnostic adequacy must perform two to four dedicated passes for cell block or obtain a core biopsy.

Pitfalls in EUS-FNA Cytology

Although encountered rarely, false-positive FNA has been reported in the literature, particularly when evaluating pancreatic diseases.[16,17] Chronic pancreatitis and auto-immune pancreatitis are the most common reasons for a false-positive diagnosis of malignancy. Some of the cytologic features that may mimic malignancy in chronic pancreatitis are occasional atypical cells, which include enlarged cells, enlarged nuclei with degenerative vacuoles, single cells, and occasional mitosis. Likewise, aspirations from autoimmune pancreatitis often show marked stromal reaction with embedded small clusters of atypical epithelial cells. It is also important to recognize that cytologic features of primary pancreatic carcinomas are similar to many other adenocarcinomas, which can metastasize to the pancreas. Immunohistochemical stains can reliably suggest the possible primary site of tumor. Therefore, it is important to perform dedicated passes to form a cell block to aid in performing immunohistochemical stains or other ancillary studies when the diagnosis is unclear.

A false-negative diagnosis may occur because of technical difficulties, sampling error, or interpretive errors. For a cytopathologist, offering diagnosis on hypocellular samples is one of the more common causes for delivering a false diagnosis. It is also possible that the marked desmoplasia of pancreatic adenocarcinoma might result in an inadequate specimen, which is commonly encountered in the setting of chronic pancreatitis.[18] Diagnosing well-differentiated adenocarcinoma can be challenging because they tend to lack the typical hyperchromasia, display minimal architectural disorder of epithelial fragments, and have only modestly increased nuclear-cytoplasmic ratios.[19] The differential diagnosis includes reactive epithelial changes, which is often associated with ductal stenting or other instrumentation. Under these circumstances, an increased number of passes may be necessary and the specimen needs to be fixed in alcohol for better delineation of nuclear morphology. Several biomarkers are increasingly available to distinguish reactive ductal epithelium from neoplastic cells. Occasionally, even a repeat EUS-FNA procedure is unrevealing and the patient may require an open surgical biopsy for histologic diagnosis.[20,21]

Whenever possible, one or more dedicated passes must be obtained for cell block creation so that, should a need arise, ancillary testing can be performed. Alternatively, a core biopsy can be performed to facilitate the same outcome.

Assessment for Molecular Markers

Enormous strides have been made in the treatment of breast and lung cancers where delivery of chemotherapeutic agents is guided by expression of molecular markers in the tumor. These molecular markers help prognosticate the tumor and guide treatment algorithm.[22,23] Despite poor clinical outcomes, treatment of pancreatic cancer has not shown much progress and available data on molecular-based treatment are primitive at best.[24–26] There is growing evidence that immune cells in pancreatic ductal adenocarcinoma produce immunosuppressive signals that allow tumors to evade the immune response.[27] Furthermore, the stromal fibroblasts provide a protective environment that not only supports and promotes pancreatic adenocarcinoma tumor growth and progression, but also likely suppresses development and/or access of antitumor immune responses. Strategies to deplete the desmoplastic stroma before immune therapy is instituted could possibly promote robust response against tumor cells. Likewise, recent studies have shown that the gene ANG2 is overexpressed in core biopsies of pancreatic neuroendocrine tumors and could potentially serve as a molecular marker or therapeutic target.[28] It is increasingly clear that the evaluation of fibrous stroma for molecular markers may become an integral part of cancer therapy.

In a recent study, specimens obtained from EUS-FNA with a 22-G needle were processed by the standard cytologic approach and compared with another cohort that were formalin fixed to preserve microcores of tissue before histologic processing.[29] EUS-FNA histology preserved the tumor tissue architecture with neoplastic glands embedded in the stroma in 67.8% of diagnostic cases compared with 27.5% with standard cytology. Furthermore, microcore samples were suitable for molecular analysis including the immunohistochemical detection of intranuclear Hes1 in malignant cells and the laser-capture microdissection-mediated measurement of Gli-1 mRNA in tumor stromal myofibroblasts.

Although data are limited, it is becoming apparent that histologic core tissue is preferred over a cytologic aspirate for assessment of molecular markers. It is also evident that the technique of specimen preservation/preparation is as important as the procedure itself. In future, we anticipate that advanced endoscopy fellows will be trained not only to procure tissue but also to assess for diagnostic adequacy and have the requisite knowledge in specimen processing, because these have important implications for patient management.

THE FUTURE OF EUS-GUIDED TISSUE ACQUISITION

Although the technique of EUS-FNA is certainly a disruptive innovation in tissue acquisition, the procedure itself continues to evolve. The pendulum has swung from histology to cytology and as evident from this discussion there is renewed interest in histology again. This interest, rational or not, is attributed to the concept that tissue cores may obtain samples with fewer needle passes, does not involve onsite specimen assessment, provides architecture, and ancillary studies can be performed on these samples. When evaluating lymphadenopathy, it is useful not only to establish a diagnosis of lymphoma but also to characterize the architecture, which is important for the diagnosis of follicular center cell lymphomas and Hodgkin lymphomas. They also could be useful in cases where flow cytometry results are false-negative, such as in large B cell lymphomas. Sections made from core biopsies are thin, 3- to 5-μm slices of tissue that when stained and viewed microscopically reveal cells or portions of cells within their intact tissue stroma. Finally, most histopathologists are very familiar and comfortable with this method of tissue-based assessment.

However, one must be aware that analysis of tissue core may not always provide a diagnosis. Needle core biopsies can pose a greater challenge in diagnosing well-differentiated pancreatic cancer in comparison with FNA samples. The inability to establish a histologic diagnosis by percutaneous techniques was one of the main reasons why EUS-guided FNA cytology rose into prominence. A major advantage of EUS-FNA cytology is that an on-site diagnosis can be established reliably in most patients and in one study the concordance between onsite and final diagnosis for malignancy was 98%.[30] However, if only core biopsies were to be performed, patients would have to wait at least 48 hours for a diagnosis. This has practical implications because consultative and diagnostic work-up may be delayed, particularly for patients traveling long distances.

To fill this vacuum, a EUS compatible Tru-Cut biopsy needle was developed nearly a decade ago but yielded suboptimal results.[31] The inherent stiffness of the 19-G platform and difficulty with the firing mechanism precluded its use for the sampling of pancreatic head and uncinate lesions. In addition, a Tru-Cut biopsy represents a single pass into the tissue and does not enable fanning, which is critical for representative sampling of lesional material. This technical limitation has now been overcome with the recent development of reverse-bevel biopsy needles (ProCore; Cook Medical, Winston-Salem, NC), which are available in multiple gauges (19-, 22-, 25-G) and do not preclude the fanning maneuver.[12] In addition, preliminary evidence suggests that a standard or Flexible 19-G needle (Expect TM Flex 19; Boston Scientific, Natick, MA) can yield histologic core tissue.[15,32] The advantages and limitations of these needles are discussed elsewhere in this issue.

There is yet no evidence that molecular marker–based treatment will improve the clinical outcomes in pancreatic cancer. There is not yet evidence that for EUS-guided tissue acquisition, histology is superior to cytology. Finally, if a cell block can be created using multiple FNA passes, do we still need histology? What is the ideal number of FNA passes that one has to perform to create an optimal cell block?

Despite the lack of clarity on multiple fronts, new accessories capable of procuring core tissue are commercially available and may be in excess of what is really needed. Critical reasoning and research is important to identify what is needed next. Ultimately, the most ideal technology or technique has to be borne out of sound reason and clinical judgment, and must impact patient care in a meaningful manner.

REFERENCES

1. Eltoum IA, Alston EA, Roberson J. Trends in pancreatic pathology practice before and after implementation of endoscopic ultrasound-guided fine-needle aspiration. Arch Pathol Lab Med 2012;136:447–53.
2. Christensen CM. The innovator's dilemma: when new technologies cause great firms to fail. Boston: Harvard Business School Press; 1997.
3. Roy A, Kim M, Hawes RH, et al. Changing trends in tissue acquisition in pancreatic diseases [abstract]. Gastrointest Endosc 2013;77:134.
4. Klapman JB, Logroño R, Dye CE, et al. Clinical impact of on-site cytopathology interpretation on endoscopic ultrasound-guided fine needle aspiration. Am J Gastroenterol 2003;98:1289–94.
5. Iglesias-Garcia J, Dominguez-Munoz JE, Abdulkader I, et al. Influence of on-site cytopathology evaluation on the diagnostic accuracy of endoscopic ultrasound-guided fine needle aspiration (EUS-FNA) of solid pancreatic masses. Am J Gastroenterol 2011;106:1705–10.
6. Alsohaibani F, Girgis S, Sandha GS. Does onsite cytotechnology evaluation improve the accuracy of endoscopic ultrasound-guided fine-needle aspiration biopsy? Can J Gastroenterol 2009;23:26–30.

7. Wani S, Mullady D, Early DS, et al. Clinical impact of immediate on-site cyto-pathology (CyP) evaluation during endoscopic ultrasound-guided fine needle aspiration (EUS-FNA) of pancreatic mass: interim analysis of a multicenter randomized controlled trial [abstract supplement]. Gastrointest Endosc 2013; 77:2.
8. Hewitt MJ, McPhail MJ, Possamai L, et al. EUS-guided FNA for diagnosis of solid pancreatic neoplasms: a meta-analysis. Gastrointest Endosc 2012;7(5):319–31.
9. Hébert-Magee S, Bae S, Varadarajulu S, et al. The presence of a cytopathologist increases the diagnostic accuracy of endoscopic ultrasound-guided fine needle aspiration cytology for pancreatic adenocarcinoma: a meta-analysis. Cytopathology 2013;24:159–71.
10. Hayashi T, Ishiwatari H, Yoshida M, et al. Rapid on-site evaluation by endosonographer during endoscopic ultrasound-guided fine needle aspiration for pancreatic solid masses. J Gastroenterol Hepatol 2013;28:656–63.
11. Masu K, Fujita N, Ito K, et al. Diagnostic efficacy of EUS-guided FNA of pancreatic masses using the cell block method without rapid on-site cytology [abstract]. Gastrointest Endosc 2013;398.
12. Iglesias-Garcia J, Poley JW, Larghi A, et al. Feasibility and yield of a new EUS histology needle: results from a multicenter, pooled, cohort study. Gastrointest Endosc 2011;73:1189–96.
13. Bang JY, Hebert-Magee S, Trevino J, et al. Randomized trial comparing the 22-gauge aspiration and 22-gauge biopsy needles for EUS-guided sampling of solid pancreatic mass lesions. Gastrointest Endosc 2012;76(2):321–7.
14. Iwashita T, Nakai Y, Samarasena JB, et al. High single-pass diagnostic yield of a new 25-gauge core biopsy needle for EUS-guided FNA biopsy in solid pancreatic lesions. Gastrointest Endosc 2013;77:909–15.
15. Larghi A, Verna EC, Ricci R, et al. EUS-guided fine-needle tissue acquisition by using a 19-gauge needle in a selected patient population: a prospective study. Gastrointest Endosc 2011;74:504–10.
16. Weynand B, Deprez P. Endoscopic ultrasound guided fine needle aspiration in biliary and pancreatic diseases: pitfalls and performances. Acta Gastroenterol Belg 2004;67:294–300.
17. Deshpande V, Mino-Kenudson M, Brugge WR, et al. Endoscopic ultrasound guided fine needle aspiration biopsy of autoimmune pancreatitis. Diagnostic criteria and pitfalls. Am J Surg Pathol 2005;29:1464–71.
18. Varadaraulu S, Tamhane A, Eloubeidi MA. Yield of EUS-guided FNA of pancreatic masses in the presence or the absence of chronic pancreatitis. Gastrointest Endosc 2005;62:728–36.
19. Kulesza P, Eltoum IA. Endoscopic ultrasound-guided fine-needle aspiration: sampling, pitfalls, and quality management. Clin Gastroenterol Hepatol 2007;5: 1248–54.
20. DeWitt J, McGreevy K, Sherman S, et al. Utility of a repeated EUS at a tertiary-referral center. Gastrointest Endosc 2008;67:610–9.
21. Eloubeidi MA, Varadarajulu S, Desai S, et al. Value of repeat endoscopic ultrasound-guided fine needle aspiration for suspected pancreatic cancer. J Gastroenterol Hepatol 2008;23:567–70.
22. Kurebayashi J, Kanomata N, Yamashita T, et al. Prognostic value of phosphorylated HER2 in HER2-positive breast cancer patients treated with adjuvant trastuzumab. Breast Cancer 2013. [Epub ahead of print].
23. Cottini F, Lautenschlaeger T. Predictors of biomarkers guiding targeted therapeutic strategies in locally advanced lung cancer. Cancer J 2013;19:263–71.

24. Maréchal R, Van Laethem JL. Towards a tailored therapy in pancreatic cancer. Acta Gastroenterol Belg 2013;76:49–56.
25. Vonderheide RH, Bajor DL, Winograd R, et al. CD40 immunotherapy for pancreatic cancer. Cancer Immunol Immunother 2013;62:949–54.
26. di Magliano MP, Logsdon CD. Roles for KRAS in pancreatic tumor development and progression. Gastroenterology 2013;144:1220–9.
27. Zheng L, Xue J, Jaffee EM, et al. Role of immune cells and immune-based therapies in pancreatitis and pancreatic ductal adenocarcinoma. Gastroenterology 2013;44:1230–40.
28. Bloomston M, Durkin A, Yang I, et al. Identification of molecular markers specific for pancreatic neuroendocrine tumors by genetic profiling of core biopsies. Ann Surg Oncol 2004;11:413–9.
29. Brais RJ, Davies SE, O'Donovan M, et al. Direct histological processing of EUS biopsies enables rapid molecular biomarker analysis for interventional pancreatic cancer trials. Pancreatology 2012;12:8–15.
30. Eloubeidi MA, Tamhane A, Jhala N, et al. Agreement between rapid onsite and final cytologic interpretations of EUS-guided FNA specimens: implications for the endosonographer and patient management. Am J Gastroenterol 2006;101:2841–7.
31. Varadarajulu S, Fraig M, Schmulewitz N, et al. Comparison of EUS-guided 19-gauge Trucut needle biopsy with EUS-guided fine-needle aspiration. Endoscopy 2004;36:397–401.
32. Varadarajulu S, Bang JY, Hebert-Magee S. Assessment of the technical performance of the flexible 19-gauge EUS-FNA needle. Gastrointest Endosc 2012;76:336–43.

Beyond Cytology
Why and When Does the Oncologist Require Core Tissue?

Sebastian G. de la Fuente, MD, J. Pablo Arnoletti, MD*

KEYWORDS

- Endoscopic ultrasound (EUS) • Fine-needle aspiration (FNA)
- Core needle biopsy (CNB) • Pancreatic cancer
- Gastrointestinal stromal tumor (GIST) • Lymphoma

KEY POINTS

- The need for core tissue to improve diagnostic accuracy and facilitate tumor and/or molecular profiling is justified in lymph node biopsy (thoracic and abdominal tumor staging; lymphomas), pancreatic and periampullary tumors, gastrointestinal stromal cell tumors, and soft tissue sarcomas.
- There are 2 main reasons why oncologists may require additional tissue and a histologic section in addition to cytopathology from fine-needle aspiration (FNA) specimens: improved diagnostic accuracy and molecular characterization of tumors.
- Rather than mutually exclusive diagnostic procedures, endoscopic ultrasound (EUS) FNA and EUS core needle biopsy (CNB) must be viewed as supplementary techniques, and both approaches should be incorporated as essential tools in the current endoscopic armamentarium.
- EUS-FNA remains the cornerstone of diagnostic biopsy procedures for upper gastrointestinal tumors, pancreatic neoplasms, and their surrounding lymph nodes.
- EUS-CNB with histologic assessment may be useful in cases such as pancreatic tumors other than pancreatic adenocarcinoma, tumors surrounded by chronic pancreatitis, submucosal and intramural gastrointestinal tumors, and for the biopsy of lesions or lymph nodes in which lymphoma is suspected.
- The added value of histologic architecture as well as thorough immunohistochemical staining may further improve diagnostic accuracy in those settings.

INTRODUCTION

Tissue acquisition is of paramount importance to confirm diagnosis and guide treatment in a wide variety of thoracic and abdominal neoplasms. In the past decade, endoscopic and minimally invasive techniques have become the procedures of

Florida Hospital Orlando, University of Central Florida, Orlando, FL, USA
* Corresponding author. 2415 North Orange Avenue, Suite 400, Orlando, FL 32804.
E-mail address: pablo.arnoletti.md@flhosp.org

Gastrointest Endoscopy Clin N Am 24 (2014) 9–17
http://dx.doi.org/10.1016/j.giec.2013.08.001
1052-5157/14/$ – see front matter © 2014 Elsevier Inc. All rights reserved.

choice to sample deep structures that could only be biopsied through open techniques in the past. The introduction of endoscopic ultrasound (EUS) has revolutionized the management of patients presenting with gastrointestinal (GI) malignancies, reaching the status of standard of care in most industrialized nations. Tumors that in the past required surgical biopsies with prolonged convalescence are now routinely accessed endoscopically, allowing expedited recovery and accelerated initiation of definitive therapies. A high sensitivity and specificity coupled with an excellent safety profile has turned EUS–fine-needle aspiration (FNA) into the preferred approach for staging mediastinal lymph node involvement in lung cancer, biopsy of pancreatic and periampullary tumors, diagnosis of submucosal tumors of the GI tract (particularly GI stromal tumors [GISTs]), and biopsy of deep-seated lymphomas. Growing experience with pancreatic and gastric tumors has allowed expansion of the indications of this approach to now include other conditions such as esophageal cancers, rectal tumors, and lung diseases. To date, EUS-guided FNA procedures offer a diagnostic accuracy of 70% to 98% depending on the location of the target lesion and experience of the operator.[1,2]

Despite current widespread availability of EUS-FNA, the technique is associated with limitations related to accessibility and interpretation of cytology samples.[3] Among the limitations of this technique, is that it only provides a cytologic specimen often with scant cellularity and, by definition, devoid of histologic architecture. EUS-FNA requires multiple needle passes and an on-site cytopathologist. Disruption of the tissue architecture during sampling of malignancies necessitating complete tissue analysis for diagnosis and grade differentiation, such as sarcomas or lymphomas, is the most notable limitation.[4–6] In addition, patients with inflammatory processes that mimic cancer pose challenges to the endoscopist and cytopathologist interpreting the results.[7–9] Furthermore, in the era of molecular profiling and personalized oncologic therapies, the need for complete histologic samples has become of paramount importance. Because of these restraints, growing interest in the use of larger caliber needles has prompted trials comparing FNA with core biopsy techniques or a combination of both.[10–17] Several studies have shown the efficacy and safety profile of EUS-guided core biopsies in a variety of different sites.[18–20] This article discusses the importance of core tissue acquisition in GI oncology, specifically focusing on upper GI and hepatopancreatobiliary conditions.

DIAGNOSIS OF PANCREATIC AND PERIAMPULLARY TUMORS

The diagnostic yield for EUS-FNA of solid pancreatic tumors ranges from 75% to 98%, with rare false-positives and a false-negative rate up to 15% in the setting of chronic pancreatitis.[21] EUS-FNA has also been proved to be helpful in the evaluation of periampullary masses that cannot be well visualized on computed tomography scan.[22] EUS core needle biopsy (CNB) seems to be a useful adjunct in those cases in which lymphoma or histology other than ductal adenocarcinoma are suspected. By providing a histologic specimen, a better microscopic examination of the tissue may be performed while providing additional tissue for immunohistochemical characterization.

Early studies have investigated the accuracy of EUS-CNB with no clear advantage compared with FNA. In a pilot study of 18 patients, 3 of whom had pancreatic masses, Varadarajulu and colleagues[17] determined the specimen adequacy and diagnostic accuracy of both techniques and concluded that there were no significant differences between EUS-CNB and EUS-FNA in diagnostic accuracy (78% vs 89%). Wittmann and colleagues[23] subsequently published their experience in 83 pancreatic patients who underwent EUS-FNA alone (lesions <2 cm) or the combination of both sampling modalities (lesions ≥2 cm). In this series, adequate samples were obtained by FNA in 94% and by CNB in 81%, compared with 87% and 92% from nonpancreatic sites (n = 76), respectively. In this study, the combination of both techniques resulted in more adequate samples from nonpancreatic cases than EUS-FNA alone (P = .044). In pancreatic cases, the investigators reported an accuracy of EUS-FNA alone of 77%; for EUS-CNB alone, 56%; and for EUS-FNA/CNB, 83%. The complication rate of this combined approach was minimal. A more recent study from the United Kingdom of 113 patients with pancreatic masses showed similar complication rates to EUS-FNA techniques.[24]

DIAGNOSIS AND CHARACTERIZATION OF GIST AND RETROPERITONEAL SOFT TISSUE SARCOMAS

EUS techniques have been increasingly used in the armamentarium of diagnostic methodologies of submucosal tumors of the GI tract. Guidelines for determination of malignancy are based on tumor size, heterogeneity of the lesion, irregularity of the borders, presence of enlarged lymph nodes, and invasion of vascular structures.[25] When FNA is added to the procedure, the sensitivity of cytologic sampling has been reported to range from 88% to 100%.[26,27] Nevertheless, in cases of suspected GIST, it may not possible to obtain features that could potentially dictate the therapeutic course of action, such as mitotic counts and immunohistochemical stains, from the cytologic sample. Because of these limitations of FNA, some investigators have explored the possibility of a 19-gauge spring-loaded EUS-CNB needle in the diagnosis of suspected GIST.[28]

DeWitt and colleagues[29] enrolled 38 consecutive patients in a prospective single-center study of patients with lesions greater than 2 cm to undergo a EUS-CNB once the on-site FNA was deemed suboptimal. In this study, EUS-CNB provided diagnostic histology and positive immunochemistry for c-kit for 79% and 97% of the patients, respectively. Based on these encouraging results, the investigators concluded that, for the initial biopsy of GIST, EUS-CNB might be considered an acceptable alternative to EUS-FNA. In contrast, in a separate European randomized crossover study, Fernández-Esparrach and colleagues[15] found that, when inadequate samples were obtained, the overall diagnostic accuracy of EUS-FNA was similar to that of EUS-CNB. Among the samples that were adequate, immunohistochemistry could be performed in 74% of EUS-FNA samples and in 91% of EUS-CNB samples (P = .025). Based on this, the investigators concluded that EUS-CNB is not superior to EUS-FNA in GISTs because of the high rate of technical failure of Tru-Cut biopsy. However, when an adequate sampling was obtained with EUS-CNB, immunohistochemical phenotyping was almost always possible. Most investigators agree that EUS-CNB is useful when immunohistochemistry is necessary[30] and previous FNA attempts have failed to provide enough tissue acquisition. The accuracy of dual sampling (EUS-CNB plus EUS-FNA) is superior to either technique alone; however, for non-transduodenal routes, the failure rate of EUS-CNB is low and the accuracy for the detection of malignancy is similar to that of EUS-FNA.[31]

With regard to the use of EUS-CNB techniques for retroperitoneal masses such as sarcomas, the data are spare and limited to case reports,[32,33] probably because, given their size, most tumors are correctly diagnosed by percutaneous core biopsy methods. The use of EUS-CNB for retroperitoneal masses could potential be applied in the future more frequently to determine tumor grade or molecular features of the mass once advances in genetic profiling become more clinically relevant.[34]

DIAGNOSIS OF DEEP-SEATED LYMPHOMAS

EUS-FNA is routinely used, with excellent sensitivity and specificity, to sample peri-intestinal lymph nodes when nodal metastases are suspected.[35–37] Despite its accuracy, diagnosis of deep-seated lymph nodes, and specifically lymphomas, can be challenging, particularly when flow cytometry is performed on the aspirated atypical lymphoid cells. In addition to tissue architecture, immunophenotype and genetic abnormalities should be assessed during diagnosis and classification of lymphoproliferative disorders. Despite the limitations inherent in EUS-FNA, investigators from Japan[38] recently reported 240 patients with suspected lymphoma who were diagnosed by EUS-FNA. Ninety-six percent of the patients were accurately diagnosed by FNA with flow cytometry showing unusual cell populations in a significant number of patients, deeming EUS-CNB unnecessary. In those patients in whom diagnostic uncertainty is present, EUS-CNB can potentially provide additional information to aid in the final diagnosis of patients with enlarged generalized lymphadenopathy.[30,39]

STAGING LYMPHATIC SPREAD OF UPPER GI, PANCREATIC, AND BILIARY TUMORS

At present, demonstration of metastatic disease to nodal tissue in upper GI, pancreatic, and biliary tumors can be provided reliably with EUS-FNA without the added need for EUS-CNB in most cases. In one of the largest series investigating EUS-FNA in the diagnosis of abdominal adenopathy, Coe and colleagues[37] showed excellent tissue acquisition even when hematopoietic disease was suspected. In this series, a sensitivity and specificity of 96% and 99%, respectively, were reported. These findings are in accordance with others,[40,41] even when mediastinal lymphadenopathy is sampled.[42]

MOLECULAR PROFILING OF TUMORS

With less than a 5% long-term survival rate, pancreatic ductal adenocarcinoma (PDAC) is almost uniformly lethal. In order to make a significant impact on the survival of patients with this malignancy, it is necessary to diagnose the disease early, when curative surgery is still possible. Detailed knowledge of the natural history of the disease and molecular events leading to its progression are therefore critical. Molecular profiling of pancreatic carcinomas is an attractive concept that continues to evolve. A major challenge to the development of biomarkers for PDAC is the small amount of tissue obtained at the time of diagnosis. EUS-FNA specimens are helpful for diagnostic purposes, but offer few additional cells for tumor characterization, and that is typically possible only in a subset of patients.[43] Furthermore, single-gene analyses may not reliably predict the biology of PDAC because of its complex molecular makeup. MicroRNA profiling may provide a more informative molecular interrogation of tumors.

Several investigators have reported the feasibility and reliability of *KRAS* gene point mutation analysis from pancreatic cancer specimens, procured by EUS-FNA, as a tool that may facilitate the diagnosis of underlying malignancy.[44] Inactivation of tumor suppressor genes has also been detected in EUS-FNA pancreatic tumor biopsies via immunohistochemistry for the p53 protein, improving the diagnostic sensitivity of this technique from 75% to 90%.[45] Mutations of other tumor suppressor genes relevant to pancreatic cancer tumorigenesis, such as *p16* and *SMAD4*, have also been successfully determined in EUS-FNA specimens.

Glycosylated proteins such as MUC are additional biomarkers often used in the characterization of pancreatic carcinoma and mucinous pancreatic neoplasms with malignant potential. MUC has been successfully detected during EUS-FNA pancreatic tumor sampling and may be incorporated in the characterization of these tumors, further increasing diagnostic accuracy.

However, these cytology-based techniques are time consuming and technically demanding. They are useful to increase the already high diagnostic accuracy of EUS-FNA in difficult cases such as well-differentiated tumors or in the presence of severe chronic pancreatitis. Adequate tumor profiling requires preservation of tissue architecture with intact epithelial and stromal compartments. A growing body of evidence points to pancreatic cancer stromal components as fundamental interactors of pancreatic carcinoma cells; promoting tumorigenesis and tumor resistance to targeted therapy.[46] A recent study compared the cytologic approach with direct formalin fixation of pancreatic EUS-FNA microcores and evaluated the potential to perform molecular biomarker analysis on that type of specimen.[47] Direct formalin fixation of pancreatic EUS-FNA microcores showed superiority in optimizing specimen suitability for molecular studies. Ability to assign a specimen to specific diagnostic categories did not differ significantly between the two techniques. However, the microcore technique was associated with decreased pathology costs and time, and provided a more reliable tissue assessment in cases with chronic pancreatitis. Histology microcores were particularly helpful in the determination of molecular marker expression such as E-cadherin, and analysis of signaling pathway activation including Notch, and phosphorylation of downstream KRAS mediators such as mitogen-activated protein kinases. The histologic approach also improved the yield of molecular techniques such as immunohistochemistry and laser-capture microdissection-mediated mRNA quantification. Although the clinical application of these biomarkers has not been completely elucidated, significant evidence points to their characterization as an important step to more effective individualized approaches to PDAC therapy.

Genomics-driven oncology is a rapidly expanding field that may soon expand personalized or precision cancer therapeutics to the routine care of patients with cancer. Tumor biopsies and tissue sampling are necessary first steps in the genomic profiling of patients who have cancer, particularly for those presenting with aggressive or metastatic tumors. EUS-CNB of tumors that are difficult to access, such as PDAC, may soon prove valuable in reliable tissue acquisition, not only for initial diagnostic purposes but also to identify molecular mechanisms of drug resistance once therapy has been instituted or in cases of tumor relapse and/or progression. In that regard, genomic profiling of serial tumor biopsies may soon become significant both before treatment (for patient stratification) and during treatment (to determine whether the therapeutic regimen is effectively modulating the target/pathway).[48]

COMPLICATIONS AND CONCERNS

EUS-CNB has been associated with a low complication rate (<1%) in spite of initial concerns about larger needle size and potential for hemorrhage.[23] Wittmann and colleagues[23] also noted that EUS-CNB performed with a Tru-Cut needle has been associated with a higher false-negative rate than EUS-FNA in the diagnostic biopsy of pancreatic tumors. However, there was a clear benefit in terms of diagnostic accuracy for the addition of EUS-CNB to FNA for nonpancreatic tumor sampling (95% vs 78%). The main limitations for the applicability of EUS-CNB include tumor size smaller than 2 cm in diameter, lesions approachable from the second part of the duodenum only, cystic lesions without an associated mass component, and uncorrected coagulopathy.

SUMMARY

There are 2 main reasons why oncologists may require additional tissue and a histologic section in addition to cytopathology from FNA specimens: improved diagnostic accuracy and molecular characterization of tumors. Rather than mutually exclusive diagnostic procedures, EUS-FNA and EUS-CNB must be viewed as supplementary techniques and both approaches should be incorporated as essential tools in the current endoscopic armamentarium.

EUS-FNA remains the cornerstone of diagnostic biopsy procedures for upper GI tumors, pancreatic neoplasms, and their surrounding lymph nodes. EUS-CNB with histologic assessment may be useful in cases such as pancreatic tumors other than pancreatic adenocarcinoma, tumors surrounded by chronic pancreatitis, submucosal and intramural GI tumors, and for the biopsy of lesions or lymph nodes in which lymphoma is suspected. The added value of histologic architecture as well as thorough immunohistochemical staining may further improve diagnostic accuracy in those settings. However, EUS-CNB may derive its most significant application in the molecular characterization of carcinomas and their supporting stroma, particularly in the case of pancreatic ductal adenocarcinoma, for which comprehensive profiling of the tumor microenvironment may soon guide patient-tailored precision therapeutic approaches.

REFERENCES

1. Hasan MK, Hawes RH. EUS-guided FNA of solid pancreas tumors. Gastrointest Endosc Clin N Am 2012;22(2):155–67, vii.
2. Bluen BE, Lachter J, Khamaysi I, et al. Accuracy and quality assessment of EUS-FNA: a single-center large cohort of biopsies. Diagn Ther Endosc 2012;2012: 139563.
3. Jhala NC, Jhala DN, Chhieng DC, et al. Endoscopic ultrasound-guided fine-needle aspiration. A cytopathologist's perspective. Am J Clin Pathol 2003;120(3): 351–67.
4. Wiersema MJ, Vilmann P, Giovannini M, et al. Endosonography-guided fine-needle aspiration biopsy: diagnostic accuracy and complication assessment. Gastroenterology 1997;112(4):1087–95.
5. Ribeiro A, Vazquez-Sequeiros E, Wiersema LM, et al. EUS-guided fine-needle aspiration combined with flow cytometry and immunocytochemistry in the diagnosis of lymphoma. Gastrointest Endosc 2001;53(4):485–91.
6. Erickson RA, Sayage-Rabie L, Beissner RS. Factors predicting the number of EUS-guided fine-needle passes for diagnosis of pancreatic malignancies. Gastrointest Endosc 2000;51(2):184–90.
7. de la Fuente SG, Ceppa EP, Reddy SK, et al. Incidence of benign disease in patients that underwent resection for presumed pancreatic cancer diagnosed by endoscopic ultrasonography (EUS) and fine-needle aspiration (FNA). J Gastrointest Surg 2010;14(7):1139–42.
8. Kanno A, Ishida K, Hamada S, et al. Diagnosis of autoimmune pancreatitis by EUS-FNA by using a 22-gauge needle based on the International Consensus Diagnostic Criteria. Gastrointest Endosc 2012;76(3):594–602.

9. Khalid A, Dewitt J, Ohori NP, et al. EUS-FNA mutational analysis in differentiating autoimmune pancreatitis and pancreatic cancer. Pancreatology 2011;11(5): 482–6.

10. Storch I, Shah M, Thurer R, et al. Endoscopic ultrasound-guided fine-needle aspiration and Trucut biopsy in thoracic lesions: when tissue is the issue. Surg Endosc 2008;22(1):86–90.

11. Cho CM, Al-Haddad M, Leblanc JK, et al. Rescue Endoscopic Ultrasound (EUS)-guided Trucut biopsy following suboptimal EUS-guided fine needle aspiration for mediastinal lesions. Gut Liver 2013;7(2):150–6.

12. Aithal GP, Anagnostopoulos GK, Kaye P. EUS-guided Trucut mural biopsies in the investigation of unexplained thickening of the esophagogastric wall. Gastrointest Endosc 2005;62(4):624–9.

13. Aithal GP, Anagnostopoulos GK, Tam W, et al. EUS-guided tissue sampling: comparison of "dual sampling" (Trucut biopsy plus FNA) with "sequential sampling" (Trucut biopsy and then FNA as required). Endoscopy 2007;39(8):725–30.

14. Shah SM, Ribeiro A, Levi J, et al. EUS-guided fine needle aspiration with and without Trucut biopsy of pancreatic masses. JOP 2008;9(4):422–30.

15. Fernández-Esparrach G, Sendino O, Sole M, et al. Endoscopic ultrasound-guided fine-needle aspiration and Trucut biopsy in the diagnosis of gastric stromal tumors: a randomized crossover study. Endoscopy 2010;42(4):292–9.

16. Kipp BR, Pereira TC, Souza PC, et al. Comparison of EUS-guided FNA and Trucut biopsy for diagnosing and staging abdominal and mediastinal neoplasms. Diagn Cytopathol 2009;37(8):549–56.

17. Varadarajulu S, Fraig M, Schmulewitz N, et al. Comparison of EUS-guided 19-gauge Trucut needle biopsy with EUS-guided fine-needle aspiration. Endoscopy 2004;36(5):397–401.

18. Mohamadnejad M, Al-Haddad MA, Sherman S, et al. Utility of EUS-guided biopsy of extramural pelvic masses. Gastrointest Endosc 2012;75(1):146–51.

19. Lee JH, Choi KD, Kim MY, et al. Clinical impact of EUS-guided Trucut biopsy results on decision making for patients with gastric subepithelial tumors >/= 2 cm in diameter. Gastrointest Endosc 2011;74(5):1010–8.

20. Chu YY, Lien JM, Ng SC, et al. Endoscopic ultrasound-guided Tru-cut biopsy for diagnosis of gastrointestinal stromal tumors. Hepatogastroenterology 2010; 57(102–103):1157–60.

21. Eloubeidi MA, Jhala D, Chhieng DC, et al. Yield of endoscopic ultrasound-guided fine-needle aspiration biopsy in patients with suspected pancreatic carcinoma. Cancer 2003;99(5):285–92.

22. Wang W, Shpaner A, Krishna SG, et al. Use of EUS-FNA in diagnosing pancreatic neoplasm without a definitive mass on CT. Gastrointest Endosc 2013;78(1):73–80.

23. Wittmann J, Kocjan G, Sgouros SN, et al. Endoscopic ultrasound-guided tissue sampling by combined fine needle aspiration and Trucut needle biopsy: a prospective study. Cytopathology 2006;17(1):27–33.

24. Thomas T, Kaye PV, Ragunath K, et al. Efficacy, safety, and predictive factors for a positive yield of EUS-guided Trucut biopsy: a large tertiary referral center experience. Am J Gastroenterol 2009;104(3):584–91.

25. Ponsaing LG, Kiss K, Loft A, et al. Diagnostic procedures for submucosal tumors in the gastrointestinal tract. World J Gastroenterol 2007;13(24):3301–10.

26. Wiech T, Walch A, Werner M. Histopathological classification of nonneoplastic and neoplastic gastrointestinal submucosal lesions. Endoscopy 2005;37(7):630–4.

27. Chang KJ, Katz KD, Durbin TE, et al. Endoscopic ultrasound-guided fine-needle aspiration. Gastrointest Endosc 1994;40(6):694–9.

28. Polkowski M, Gerke W, Jarosz D, et al. Diagnostic yield and safety of endoscopic ultrasound-guided Trucut [corrected] biopsy in patients with gastric submucosal tumors: a prospective study. Endoscopy 2009;41(4):329–34.

29. DeWitt J, Emerson RE, Sherman S, et al. Endoscopic ultrasound-guided Trucut biopsy of gastrointestinal mesenchymal tumor. Surg Endosc 2011;25(7): 2192–202.

30. Saftoiu A, Vilmann P, Guldhammer Skov B, et al. Endoscopic ultrasound (EUS)-guided Trucut biopsy adds significant information to EUS-guided fine-needle aspiration in selected patients: a prospective study. Scand J Gastroenterol 2007;42(1):117–25.

31. Polkowski M, Larghi A, Weynand B, et al. Learning, techniques, and complications of endoscopic ultrasound (EUS)-guided sampling in gastroenterology: European Society of Gastrointestinal Endoscopy (ESGE) technical guideline. Endoscopy 2012;44(2):190–206.

32. Gill KR, Hasan MK, Menke DM, et al. Presacral myelolipoma: diagnosis by EUS-FNA and Trucut biopsy. Gastrointest Endosc 2010;71(4):849 [discussion: 849–50].

33. Kalapala R, Lakhtakia S, Reddy DN. Endoscopic ultrasonography-guided core biopsy diagnosis of giant adrenal myelolipoma. Clin Gastroenterol Hepatol 2012;10(4):e36–7.

34. Italiano A, Lagarde P, Brulard C, et al. Genetic profiling identifies two classes of soft-tissue leiomyosarcomas with distinct clinical characteristics. Clin Cancer Res 2013;19(5):1190–6.

35. Eloubeidi MA, Wallace MB, Reed CE, et al. The utility of EUS and EUS-guided fine needle aspiration in detecting celiac lymph node metastasis in patients with esophageal cancer: a single-center experience. Gastrointest Endosc 2001; 54(6):714–9.

36. Levy MJ, Jondal ML, Clain J, et al. Preliminary experience with an EUS-guided Trucut biopsy needle compared with EUS-guided FNA. Gastrointest Endosc 2003;57(1):101–6.

37. Coe A, Conway J, Evans J, et al. The yield of EUS-FNA in undiagnosed upper abdominal adenopathy is very high. J Clin Ultrasound 2013;41(4):210–3.

38. Yasuda I, Goto N, Tsurumi H, et al. Endoscopic ultrasound-guided fine needle aspiration biopsy for diagnosis of lymphoproliferative disorders: feasibility of immunohistological, flow cytometric, and cytogenetic assessments. Am J Gastroenterol 2012;107(3):397–404.

39. Eloubeidi MA, Mehra M, Bean SM. EUS-guided 19-gauge Trucut needle biopsy for diagnosis of lymphoma missed by EUS-guided FNA. Gastrointest Endosc 2007;65(6):937–9.

40. Nakahara O, Yamao K, Bhatia V, et al. Usefulness of endoscopic ultrasound-guided fine needle aspiration (EUS-FNA) for undiagnosed intra-abdominal lymphadenopathy. J Gastroenterol 2009;44(6):562–7.

41. Yasuda I, Tsurumi H, Omar S, et al. Endoscopic ultrasound-guided fine-needle aspiration biopsy for lymphadenopathy of unknown origin. Endoscopy 2006; 38(9):919–24.

42. Chen VK, Eloubeidi MA. Endoscopic ultrasound-guided fine needle aspiration is superior to lymph node echofeatures: a prospective evaluation of mediastinal and peri-intestinal lymphadenopathy. Am J Gastroenterol 2004;99(4): 628–33.

43. Arnoletti JP, Frolov A, Eloubeidi M, et al. A phase I study evaluating the role of the anti-epidermal growth factor receptor (EGFR) antibody cetuximab as a

radiosensitizer with chemoradiation for locally advanced pancreatic cancer. Cancer Chemother Pharmacol 2011;67(4):891–7.

44. Kato K, Kamada H, Fujimori T, et al. Molecular biologic approach to the diagnosis of pancreatic carcinoma using specimens obtained by EUS-guided fine needle aspiration. Gastroenterol Res Pract 2012;2012:243524.

45. Itoi T, Takei K, Sofuni A, et al. Immunohistochemical analysis of p53 and MIB-1 in tissue specimens obtained from endoscopic ultrasonography-guided fine needle aspiration biopsy for the diagnosis of solid pancreatic masses. Oncol Rep 2005; 13(2):229–34.

46. Liles JS, Arnoletti JP, Kossenkov AV, et al. Targeting ErbB3-mediated stromal-epithelial interactions in pancreatic ductal adenocarcinoma. Br J Cancer 2011; 105(4):523–33.

47. Brais RJ, Davies SE, O'Donovan M, et al. Direct histological processing of EUS biopsies enables rapid molecular biomarker analysis for interventional pancreatic cancer trials. Pancreatology 2012;12(1):8–15.

48. Garraway LA. Genomics-driven oncology: framework for an emerging paradigm. J Clin Oncol 2013;31(15):1806–14.

Definitions in Tissue Acquisition
Core Biopsy, Cell Block, and Beyond

Nirag Jhala, MD, MIAC[a],*, Darshana Jhala, MD, BMus[b]

KEYWORDS

- Direct smears • Cell block • Needle core biopsy • Fine-needle aspiration
- Endoscopic ultrasound • Cytology

KEY POINTS

- A successful cytology practice mandates teamwork and close interaction between a skillful tissue procurer and an experienced cytopathologist.
- The goal of cytologic preparation is to obtain the representative cells in an appropriate and optimum state for microscopic examination; without too much overlapping or too much spreading of the cells over a large area.
- Many different staining protocols have been used in cytology practices.
- Cell blocks should always be used in conjunction with analysis of smears and other cytologic preparations.
- Telepathology has rapidly evolved from a simple model of capture, store, and forward concept of static images to a very complex and dynamic process, which holds promise to significantly change the way anatomic pathology is being practiced today.

INTRODUCTION

Fine-needle aspiration (FNA) and small-tissue sampling and analysis are complex and highly coordinated processes. The main objective of tissue sampling of a focal lesion by endoscopic ultrasonography (EUS)-guided fine-needle aspiration biopsy (FNAB) and/or core-needle biopsy (CNB) is to provide a rapid, accurate, and cost-efficient diagnosis for informed decision making and appropriate patient management. Samples obtained using these modalities, however, should be handled with care because whichever modality is used (FNA or CNB), the samples procured are limited in volume. The main components required to optimize cell yield are interlinked with each other, and include (1) sample acquisition, (2) sample handling and preparation, and (3) analysis. A preliminary understanding of how samples are prepared for cytology

[a] Department of Pathology and Laboratory Medicine, University of Pennsylvania, Philadelphia, PA 19104, USA; [b] Department of Pathology and Laboratory Medicine, Philadelphia Veterans Affairs Medical Center, University of Pennsylvania, Philadelphia, PA, USA
* Corresponding author.
E-mail address: Jhalan@uphs.upenn.edu

Gastrointest Endoscopy Clin N Am 24 (2014) 19–27
http://dx.doi.org/10.1016/j.giec.2013.08.005
1052-5157/14/$ – see front matter © 2014 Elsevier Inc. All rights reserved.

and histology, as noted in **Table 1**, would help in understanding the differences between the types of assessments offered by 2 relatively different tissue-processing methodologies. Aspirates are routinely handled as cytologic specimens; however, cell blocks and micro biopsies can be simultaneously prepared from the FNAB material for histologic examination. From core biopsies, one can obtain touch imprints for cytologic assessment as well.

A successful cytology practice mandates teamwork and close interaction between a skillful tissue procurer and an experienced cytopathologist.

SAMPLE ACQUISITION

Before other sections highlight types of needs and core biopsies, it is important to understand some differences in these terminologies.

Fine-Needle Aspiration

Aspiration of tissue sample with a needle size smaller than 21 gauge is considered as a fine-needle aspiration. For the purposes of EUS, for a long time 22-gauge, 25-gauge, and now 27-gauge needles have been used to obtain samples from various organ sites.[1–3] Using such thin needles have proved to be less invasive, and has the advantage of obtaining adequate samples from target lesions to provide an accurate diagnosis. By comparison, larger-bore needles (19-gauge) have often been used to obtain samples. Such needles offer less flexibility and are associated with greater tissue trauma. This type of sampling offers acquisition of cytology as well as micro biopsy samples.

Core-Needle Biopsy

Core biopsy needles allow acquisition of tissue core biopsies. Innovation has allowed acquisition of core biopsy samples with a needle size as small as 25-gauge, 22-gauge, and 19-gauge.[4,5] A sample acquired using this modality offers core biopsies and the advantage of reviewing tissue architecture. Such a sample often helps to reduce the number of passes. It also helps general surgical pathologists who are more familiar with such samples to render their opinions. This modality, however, is more morbid

	Cytology Technique	Histology Technique
Table 1		
Salient differences between cytology and histology processes		
Fixation	Air drying Ethanol	10% Neutral buffered formalin
Transport	Special medium for liquid-based sample processing (eg, Preservecyt, SurePath, ThinPrep, Hanks balanced salt solution)	Saline, formalin
Processing	Direct smear/centrifugation related preparations/liquid-based preparations	Gross examination Tissue processing Paraffin embedding Microtome sectioning
Staining	Papanicolaou/Romanowsky stains	Hematoxylin-eosin (H&E)
Product	Smears and liquid-based preparations: whole cells are analyzed Cell-block preparations: H&E-stained sections are analyzed	Sections (part of cells)

and may lead to an increased number of adverse events. It is recognized that cutting needles provide long, adequate samples without fragmentation. Large-bore aspiration-type needles may occasionally lead to tissue fragmentation. The moving and cutting mechanics of the various large-bore needles underlie the procurement of the tissue samples, which often include tumor and host tissue as well.

In view of the differences, the 2 modalities (FNA and CNB) complement each other when performed at the same sitting.

Key Features: Sample Acquisition

- The operator is the most important team member, whose task is to provide representative and sufficient samples.
- The fundamentals for successful aspiration are negative pressure, precision, and intralesional placement of the needle at all times when negative pressure is applied.
- The fundamentals for successful core biopsy are needle type and moving mechanics, precision, and positioning of the needle in the vicinity and into the mass.
- Route of acquisition may be the source of contaminants picked up en route that may influence interpretation.

HANDLING A CYTOLOGY SAMPLE

The goal of cytologic preparation is to harvest the representative cells in an appropriate and optimum state for microscopic examination, without too much overlapping or too much spreading of the cells over a large area.

Direct smears can be sourced from aspirates and touch imprints. Direct smears can be made either by gently spreading the material using another spreader slide, or via a butterfly technique whereby samples are spread on both slides. Generally touch imprints are made from core biopsies to assess adequacy. Cellularity in touch preparations will depend on the type of lesion and the force applied to the cores when touched on the slides.

Handling of Cytology Samples

The factors involved in proper handling of cytology samples are (1) appropriate fixation, (2) appropriate number of slides, and (3) appropriate handling of excess blood.

Appropriate fixation
Wet fixation Smears still wet should be directly immersed using 95% ethanol fixative, which can be achieved by immersing slides in alcohol, placing alcohol on slides laid on a plane surface, or spraying the smears using spray fixatives. Such preparations are usually stained using Papanicolaou stain. Air drying of cells when one uses this protocol will lead to lack of staining characteristics for cells.

Dry fixation The air-dried preparation requires the cytologic smears to be immediately dried. Here, air drying serves as a fixation. In general, these slides are stained with Romanowsky stains. In instances where the smears are still wet, staining will be uneven and will lose crisp cellular details.

Appropriate number of slides
The number of slides prepared should correspond to the volume of the aspirates. There are 4 smearing methods: leveling, pushing (butterfly, facing), sliding, and crushing.

Leveling is performed when the volume of the aspirate is merely sufficient for only one slide.

Pushing is good for lymph node aspirates and granular cytologic samples. A drop of sample is expressed onto the center of the slide, and another slide is placed on it such that the material on the slide spreads by capillary action from the center to the periphery.

Sliding is more appropriate for aspirates with some fluid or for large-volume samples. If the sample is voluminous and 1 pair of slides would result in thick smears, 2 pairs or more are recommended, by dividing the samples using another opposing slide and repeating the sliding method for the divided samples.

The crushing method has to be avoided at all costs.

Appropriate handling of excess blood

Blood clots usually trap and hide the incriminating cells. One suggestion is to remove the blood clot before making the smears. Cell blocks should be prepared if there is substantial admixed tissue.

It cannot be overemphasized that sample preparation holds the key to the success of FNAB interpretation. Making a direct smear on site is one of the most basic steps that should be learned by any practitioner of cytopathology. Practice makes perfect.

Potential Pitfalls

- When aspirating from vascular organs, often there will be a significant amount of blood within the needle. In such instances, once a drop of material is placed on the slide, the sample may be concentrated with a syringe and needle to avoid making too many slides with cells entrapped in clotted blood, making them uninterpretable.
- One should also avoid the use of force while making smears, as this may lead to shearing of cells. Such smears will demonstrate many naked hyperchromatic nuclei with prominent nucleoli.

Liquid-Based Technologies

Liquid-based methodologies for preparing samples use either membrane filter or cyto-centrifugation. The former uses membranes with pores small enough to filter out fluid and debris. The cells are captured on the membrane that is transparent under light microscopy. The latter basically uses centrifugation to concentrate cells in a limited area. These techniques are suitable for cytologic samples, collected in liquid. The most significant benefit over conventional cytology is the even fixation and preparation.

Cytospin and Millipore filter are 2 basic methods still performed in laboratories for liquid-based samples. These methods are useful for needle rinses and cyst contents. Cytospin, the trade name for cytocentrifugation, offers concentrated samples placed in a defined area on a slide, thereby improving cell yield as well as providing evenly distributed cells. Millipore membrane filters are made of biologically inert mixtures of cellulose acetate and cellulose nitrate, and serve as sieves. The advantage of these membranes is that they help to enrich cells on the membrane while allowing passage of very small particles to be eliminated from cytologic evaluation.

In recent years newer modalities of liquid-based commercial technologies, such as ThinPrep and SurePath, have been replacing older technologies. Their usage in nongynecologic cytology is gradually expanding. These different features might affect the cellular details and, hence, influence the interpretation. **Table 2** highlights salient differences between these 2 technologies.

Table 2 Comparison of 2 liquid-based technologies for nongynecologic samples		
	ThinPrep	**SurePath**
	Membrane filtration Methanol-based fixative	Cell washing and concentration on gravity sedimentation onto a coated slide Ethanol-based fixative
Technical highlights	More expensive One sample at a time	48 samples at once
Cytologic highlights	Red blood cells/crystals/bile/fat/ mucin eliminated Less overlap Flatter sheets Large sheets less prominent	More 3-dimensional structures Architecture preserved

In general with liquid-based cytology, cells tend to shrink, cell clusters fragment, papillary structures break, there are more single cells giving the impression of apparent increased cell dyscohesion, the chromatin details are changed, and nucleoli become more conspicuous. Other features such as background matrix and necrosis will be substantially reduced. Unless cytopathologists become familiar with such changes, there is a potential to err on such sample preparations. Once familiarity with this sample type is achieved, it can become a very valuable mode of preparation for analysis of FNA samples.

Disadvantages include: (1) no on-site assessment of adequacy (unless split-sample method or double-aspiration protocol is used); (2) no triage of specimens; (3) no air-dried smears for Romanowsky stains; (4) semiautomated processing but longer preparation time; (5) removal of background elements; and (6) high cost. Moreover, (7) familiarity with cytologic artifacts and recognition of diagnostic pitfalls are essential in avoiding misinterpretations.

Chromatin details, nucleoli, and intranuclear inclusions are more crystallized; however, these fine details are appreciable only in cells that are monolayered and can, in fact, be somewhat disconcerting. Cell blocks of reasonable quality can be prepared from liquid-based specimens; however, the integrity of the trabecular-sinusoidal arrangement is compromised.

On the other hand, owing to the differences in the SurePath preparatory method, background material is more likely to be retained. There is greater cellularity with preservation of architectural features, but this occurs alongside crowding and more 3-dimensional groupings, requiring much fine focusing in different planes to unravel any informative features.

Immunocytochemistry can be successfully applied to thin-layer cytology slides. However, just as in conventional smears, the 3-dimensional aspect of cell clusters may obscure finer details.

Staining
Many different staining protocols have been used in cytology practices. There are 2 main categories of conventional stains.

Romanowsky stains Modifications of Romanowsky stains are used in different laboratories for the assessment of cytology samples; for example, DiffQuik and May-Grün-wald Giemsa (MGG). DiffQuik stain is technically less demanding and can be rapidly performed, hence providing rapid on-site assessment of specimen adequacy. Air drying is an important step in staining direct smears with DiffQuik. The stain itself uses 2 basic parts: Solution I is a buffered solution of Eosin Y (an anionic dye), and Solution II is composed of a buffered solution of thiazine dyes (cationic dyes) consisting of Methylene Blue and Azure A. The resultant basophilic staining of nucleoli and cytoplasm is due to the Methylene Blue component of the mixture. The anionic component of the nucleoli and cytoplasm, which is stained with the cationic Methylene Blue, is presumed to be RNA. The nuclei are stained red to purple (metachromatically) by the Azure A component of the dye mixture.

Papanicolaou stain Since the first documentation by George Papanicolaou in 1942, this stain has seen multiple modifications. It is a progressive and differential stain that generally uses 5 dyes in 3 solutions. The color reaction depends on the type of dyes used in the Papanicolaou stain. It uses hematoxylin as nuclear stain, with 2 counterstains (orange G and Eosin Azure or EA). Eosin Azure contains Eosin Y, Light green or Fast green, and Bismarck Brown. These dyes allow various colors that are noted in different cells, and provide a better delineation of nuclear details in comparison with DiffQuik stain.

As a general rule, this stain requires fixation in alcohol followed by multiple steps to provide a very crisp stain that characterizes cytoplasmic as well as nuclear details. To decrease the time needed to stain direct smears, a modification of the technique (ultrafast Pap stain) allows for rapid staining of cells after air drying. Taking only 90 seconds, the ultrafast Pap stain offers a unique advantage of staining cells on site with the Papanicolaou method, an enormous benefit for services that pride themselves on providing point-of-care testing.

Key Features: Handling of Cytology Samples

- Fixation and smearing methods are of utmost importance in providing excellent smears.
- Wet-fixed preparation is immediate immersion of the slides in 95% ethanol; the slides are stained according to Papanicolaou staining protocol.
- The smearing method most often used is the sliding method; any blood clot is first removed and the number of smeared slides prepared according to the volume of the aspirates.
- Air-dried preparation is immediate drying of smears, preferably monolayered cells; the slides are stained by DiffQuik and MGG (so-called Romanowsky stains).
- Liquid-based techniques help to enhance fixation and concentrate the cells. The preparations may influence cell morphology and affect smear background.

HANDLING A HISTOLOGY SAMPLE
Cell Blocks

Cell blocks should always be used in conjunction with analysis of smears and other cytologic preparations. These blocks provide general architecture to cells and, hence, recapitulate morphology noted on tissue sections. Because they are paraffin-embedded samples cut at thickness of 3 to 5 μm, multiple sections can be cut. Apart from the routine hematoxylin-eosin staining, the sections can be stained by special stains (histochemical, immunohistochemical, or molecular) to diagnose, distinguish, prognosticate, or predict therapeutic response. When one considers performing immunohistochemical stains, cell-block preparations offer an advantage over other cell preparations such as alcohol-fixed smears and liquid-based cytology samples.

There are several cell-block preparatory methods, each offering their unique advantages. Cellularity in cell blocks has always remained a subject of intense exploration. There are number of different ways to improve cell yield. Simple steps include (1) collection of samples in low-volume fixative/transport medium, (2) scraping of cells from direct smears after providing specimen adequacy, (3) retrieval of cells from needle hub to make a cell block, (4) placement of at least 1 and preferably 2 dedicated passes into formalin fixative after specimen adequacy has been rendered, and (5) use of cell-capturing gels, such as fibrin, Cellient technology, or histogels.

Key Features: Handling of Histology Samples

- Fixation and cell blocks are crucial to the provision of optimal histologic sections.
- 10% neutral buffered formalin is used as fixative.
- Core tissue samples should be placed on a piece of paper, and fragmented samples should be wrapped up before putting in fixatives; transit time should be as short as possible.
- Cell blocks are easily prepared and processed using a routine histology technique.
- Immunohistochemistry is easier to perform and to interpret on histologic sections.

TELEPATHOLOGY AND TELECYTOLOGY
Telepathology

Simply stated, telepathology is about practicing pathology from a distance by pathologists. Telepathology has rapidly evolved from a simple model of capture, store, and forward concept of static images to a very complex and dynamic process, which holds promise to significantly change the way anatomic pathology is being practiced today. There are various formats under which telepathology systems are being developed, including preparation of whole-slide images or images generated and dynamically transmitted over high-speed lines with operators at each end, or robot-controlled motorized light microscopes.[6,7]

Virtual slides using whole-slide scanning
As the name implies, the entire tissue on the glass slide (histopathology or cytopathology) is scanned with creation of a digital image, which is then viewed using a slide viewer. The process of slide digitization involves a series of steps, each contributing to the quality of the final image displayed on the computer screen. The steps that can affect the quality of the final image are: preimaging processes, such as sample preparation and staining; optical image acquisition by the sensor (eg, camera); formation of image by a virtual slide scanner; postprocessing of the digital information; image compression; transmission of the digital image file across a telecommunication network; and display of the digital image file on the pathologist's video display.[7] Although the underlying process of image acquisition differs, these slide scanners have over a period of time offered faster scanning speeds and higher image quality. Images can be captured at different magnifications, and algorithms are being developed to make virtual slides ever more user-friendly.

In the context of pathology services, virtual slides or whole-slide imaging systems have been used for primary diagnosis, consultative second opinions, educational purposes for teaching students at every level, developing quality-assurance parameters, developing examination files, and storage of slides on the server, which has the potential to reduce or eliminate the need for storage of actual glass slides. Although these considerations make whole-slide imaging and virtual slides very attractive, they are subject to several technique-related challenges. One of the major challenges on the user end has remained cytopathology smears with 3-dimensional perspective. These systems are continually being improved to accommodate for lacunae in the areas of image capture, stitching images, image transmission, and image-storing capability of servers. This format holds considerable promise for the future of histopathology and cytopathology.

Furthermore, image systems are increasingly incorporating concepts that have been used for years, such as DNA quantification, as well as quantifying and analyzing immunohistochemistry profiles in the hopes of providing an objective analysis. In addition, algorithms have been developed for multispectral image analysis that uses both spatial and spectral images to classify 2 similar images. Such analysis has the potential to differentiate morphologically similar lesions.

Real-time telepathology systems

These systems allow images captured on the light microscope by a high-speed camera to be transmitted in real time through a dedicated high-speed cable network over the Internet to the host computer equipped with high-end video cards. In this telecytopathology format, a cytotechnologist, advanced trainee, or fellow colleague can handle the transmission of image from the microscope and stay in direct communication with the pathologist at the other end. Another technology is "robot stage" whereby the operator for slide review can control the stage of the microscope remotely. These telecytopathology systems are better suited for facilitating on-site assessments of specimen adequacy.

In the authors' hands, on-site adequacy reported by telecytopathology compared well with on-site cytopathology evaluation (concordance rates of 88%–98%) as well as final cytologic interpretation.[8,9] These samples, however, should be interpreted with caution, as lack of color correction and image pixilation can serve as confounding factors. In addition, cellular groups may be difficult to visualize in such systems.

Key Features: Telepathology and Telecytology

- Telepathology education, consultation, and on-site service setups are promising.
- Small samples (histologic sections) are good candidates for whole scanning and image acquisition.
- Cytologic smears need more sophisticated image-acquisition techniques to cover 3-dimensional subjects.
- Real-time telepathology is ideal for rapid on-site consultation for specimen adequacy.

REFERENCES

1. Bang JY, Hebert-Magee S, Trevino J, et al. Randomized trial comparing the 22-gauge aspiration and 22-gauge biopsy needles for EUS-guided sampling of solid pancreatic mass lesions. Gastrointest Endosc 2012;76(2):321–7. PubMed PMID: 22658389.
2. Lee JH, Stewart J, Ross WA, et al. Blinded prospective comparison of the performance of 22-gauge and 25-gauge needles in endoscopic ultrasound-guided fine needle aspiration of the pancreas and peri-pancreatic lesions. Dig Dis Sci 2009; 54(10):2274–81. PubMed PMID: 19669880.
3. Vilmann P, Saftoiu A, Hollerbach S, et al. Multicenter randomized controlled trial comparing the performance of 22 gauge versus 25 gauge EUS-FNA needles in solid masses. Scand J Gastroenterol 2013;48(7):877–83. PubMed PMID: 23795663.

4. Varadarajulu S, Bang JY, Hebert-Magee S. Assessment of the technical performance of the flexible 19-gauge EUS-FNA needle. Gastrointest Endosc 2012; 76(2):336–43. PubMed PMID: 22817786.

5. Varadarajulu S, Fraig M, Schmulewitz N, et al. Comparison of EUS-guided 19-gauge Trucut needle biopsy with EUS-guided fine-needle aspiration. Endoscopy 2004;36(5):397–401. PubMed PMID: 15100946.

6. Collins BT. Telepathology in cytopathology: challenges and opportunities. Acta Cytol 2013;57(3):221–32. PubMed PMID: 23635868.

7. Pantanowitz L, Valenstein PN, Evans AJ, et al. Review of the current state of whole slide imaging in pathology. J Pathol Inform 2011;2:36. PubMed PMID: 21886892. PubMed Central PMCID: 3162745.

8. Goyal A, Jhala N, Gupta P. TeleCyP (Telecytopathology): real-time fine-needle aspiration interpretation. Acta Cytol 2012;56(6):669–77. PubMed PMID: 23207446.

9. Buxbaum JL, Eloubeidi MA, Lane CJ, et al. Dynamic telecytology compares favorably to rapid onsite evaluation of endoscopic ultrasound fine needle aspirates. Dig Dis Sci 2012;57(12):3092–7. PubMed PMID: 22729624. Pubmed Central PMCID: 3640867.

How Can an Endosonographer Assess for Diagnostic Sufficiency and Options for Handling the Endoscopic Ultrasound-Guided Fine-Needle Aspiration Specimen and Ancillary Studies

Shantel Hébert-Magee, MD

KEYWORDS

- Endoscopic ultrasound-guided fine-needle aspiration • Assessment • Adequacy
- Handling • Processing • Ancillary studies

KEY POINTS

- A basic knowledge of cytopathology is imperative for endosonographers who attempt to achieve a greater than 95% diagnostic accuracy with their tissue-acquisition procedures.
- This information is relevant for both newly established and existing endoscopic ultrasonography centers to improve their clinical outcomes and practice patterns.

INTRODUCTION

Endoscopic ultrasound-guided fine-needle aspiration (EUS-FNA) has been well established as a minimally invasive technique in diagnosing and staging various gastrointestinal, pancreaticobiliary, and retroperitoneal malignancies.[1–5] In experienced hands the diagnostic yield can be high; however, the success of EUS-FNA depends not only on the skill of the endosonographer but also on the combined effort of the endosonographer and cytopathologist working together as a functional team.[6,7] Immediate, on-site cytopathology support increases diagnostic accuracy by assessing sample adequacy, insuring proper sample processing, obviating additional unnecessary passes, and determining if additional material is required for ancillary testing.[8,9] Despite the benefits that rapid interpretation and early clinical management can have on patient care, on-site cytopathology interpretation is not available in many centers. Cost-benefit analysis and/or better use of the time of the cytopathologist or skilled cytotechnologist for other responsibilities have led to specimen handling and collection being performed by endoscopy nurses and

Department of Pathology, University of Alabama at Birmingham, Birmingham, AL 35233, USA
E-mail address: shebertm@uab.edu

Gastrointest Endoscopy Clin N Am 24 (2014) 29–56
http://dx.doi.org/10.1016/j.giec.2013.08.002
1052-5157/14/$ – see front matter © 2014 Elsevier Inc. All rights reserved.

giendo.theclinics.com

suite attendants. This article is intended to assist the independent endosonographer in the assessment of diagnostic sufficiency and in specimen handling.

FNA PREREQUISITES

Before handling the specimen, the endosonographer must have a protocol for preparation. It must be determined whether cytopathology laboratory assistance will be provided on site or if a diagnosis will be given from the laboratory on receipt of specimens. Sometimes the laboratory is not in close proximity to the procedural area, and the endosonographer may function independently until laboratory support arrives. Even in large academic centers where cytopathology assistance is readily available, the FNA procedure can occur after hours when laboratory personnel are not accessible. Therefore, if functioning independently on any level, the endosonographer must be aware of the necessary supplies and equipment needed for proper handling of the cellular materials obtained.

On-Site Evaluation

If on-site evaluation is possible, the procedural suite often has an area dedicated to specimen handling. This area usually consists of a table or mobile cart containing the equipment and materials needed for the processing and assessment of the sample. The space is often compartmentalized with a smearing and staining setup and a microscope for preliminary evaluation. The table or mobile cart also has collection tubes with varying media for ancillary studies if warranted.

Deferring to Laboratory Evaluation

Depending on the unique established protocol set up at the EUS center (**Fig. 1**) in alignment with the cytopathology laboratory, handling of the specimen can vary.

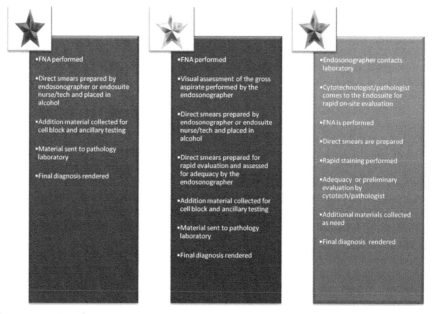

Fig. 1. Examples of tissue-handling protocols used by different EUS centers. The presence of on-site cytopathology is the preferred gold standard.

Some centers do not have capabilities for rapid assessment; therefore, needle rinsing of the cellular aspirate into media has been standard. In other centers, the endosonographer or support staff prepares the direct smears and transports them to the laboratory along with any additional materials collected for further evaluation (cell block, flow cytometry, or tumor markers).

Support Staff

To ensure proper handling and processing of the aspirated material, one must recognize the limitations and varying skills of the support staff. Although having an experienced cytopathologist on site is optimal, it may be impractical. If trained properly, a skilled technician or endoscopy nurse can prepare direct smears and crudely gauge whether cellular material is present by gross visual assessment.[10,11] However, for adequate evaluation a proficient cytotechnologist or an endosonographer with basic cytomorphology training needs to visualize the sample macroscopically and microscopically.[12,13]

Supplies Needed

A box of clean glass slides should be readily available. Frosted single-end microscope slides are suggested for FNA smear preparation, as they provide a designated labeling area and sufficient space for spreading the aspirated material. Although fully frosted slides offer greater surface adhesion, they are not recommended because of increased risk of cell distortion. Blank or plain glass slides can also be used; however, a diamond-point glass scriber is needed. For frosted single-end slides a soft lead pencil is suggested for labeling, as many "permanent" markers are not truly indelible.

For on-site evaluation at most institutions, air-dried and alcohol-fixed smears are prepared to obtain a wider range of diagnostic information. For assessment of sample adequacy and rapid interpretation, Romanowsky-type staining (Diff-Quik, Three-Step, Quik-Dip) is usually performed. The Romanowsky-type staining kits consist of a fixative, an acidophilic dye for cytoplasmic staining, and a basophilic dye for nuclear staining. Hematoxylin and eosin stains (H&E), the rapid protocol used for frozen-section evaluation, can also be performed for rapid cytologic interpretation. Alcohol-fixed smears for Papanicolaou staining must be wet-fixed and placed into 95% alcohol. Plastic Coplin jars are often used for easy transport to the cytopathology laboratory. The choice of stains used is based on institutional preferences and operator experience.[14] It has been well established in the literature that wet-fixed smears stained with H&E or Papanicolaou stain allow for better visualization of 3-dimensional clusters and nuclear detail, whereas Romanowsky-type stains tend to better highlight cytoplasmic features and extracellular substances.[15,16]

In addition to slides, marking apparatus, and staining solutions, carrying solutions (fixatives and preservatives) must be available for needle washing. As previously mentioned, some centers solely rely on needle washing. Experience has shown that watery, bloody, and mucoid samples can all make it difficult for untrained personnel to prepare adequate smears. Personnel who do not routinely make smears may encounter difficulties in preparing smears from these aspirates. Therefore, directly rinsing the aspirate into the desired carrying solution avoids the consequences of poorly smeared slides and specimen handling. Materials collected from needle rinsing can be used for direct smears, cytospin smears, cell-block preparation, flow cytometry, and other ancillary studies. The independent endosonographer must be aware of the types of solution for rinsing, as the choice of carrying media may restrict the type of processing or ancillary testing option performed. To maximize the amount of material collected, a 10-mL syringe filled with air should be used to flush any residual material from the needle.

Following universal precautions, gloves must be used when handling the aspirate.[17] Barrier gowns and masks may be warranted for patients in isolation. In addition, disposable bench-liner pads should be used for slide preparation to prevent contamination of the work area from aspirate splatter.

Ancillary Studies and Processing

Ancillary techniques have become a pertinent component in the diagnostic arm of EUS-FNA.[18-26] The information gained may have significant diagnostic and therapeutic implications that may not be available by microscopic examination. The following are some of the frequently used techniques for the diagnostic workup of aspirated material.

Immunocytochemistry

Immunocytochemistry (ICC) is usually used in the diagnostic regimen when morphology alone cannot identify or specify the pathologic process, or when markers can provide specific information for therapeutic response and/or prognosis. Immunocytochemistry is a laboratory technique that relies on antibody-antigen interaction, whereby staining is noted when antibody markers interact with antigens present in the tissue. Rarely are diagnoses rendered using a single marker, because of cross-reactivity and limitations of sensitivity and specificity; most diagnoses require an ICC panel.[27] ICC staining can easily be performed on unstained fresh smears (alcohol fixed or air-dried) and cell blocks. Cell blocks are preferable for ICC staining, because the thin sections prevent background staining, and a good cell block with ample material can allow for multiple sections (extensive panels) when needed. Using fresh EUS-FNA smears limits the number of antibody markers that can be tested, and there is a higher likelihood of background staining, which can be problematic for interpretation. Finally, most clinical immunohistochemistry laboratory protocols are optimized for formalin-fixed paraffin-embedded tissue. Whichever specimen is used, the success of ICC staining is highly dependent on the preservation of the aspirated material. If the cellular smear is left to air-dry for a significant amount of time, the desiccation process will lead to cell disruption. Similarly, if the aspirated material for cell block is not placed into a proper fixative, cell fragmentation and necrosis will occur and antigen specificity may be lost.

Microbiology

If there is a suspicion for microbial organisms in the cellular materials collected, special stains can be used. Special stains can readily identify fungi, mycobacteria, and some other microbes; however, other microorganisms may require cultures and polymerase chain reaction (PCR) for detection and speciation. Many clinical microbiology laboratories are using PCR much more frequently because of its high diagnostic accuracy, low contamination risk, and speed as an alternative to cultures for diagnosing many infectious diseases. If the sample is going to microbiology, it cannot be placed in a fixative if the culture method will be used for identification; the cells must be viable. The time between collection of the material and the initiation of the culturing process may significantly affect test results. If a delay is anticipated, an additive solution or culture medium may be needed. PCR can be performed on specimens collected in saline, cell media, and formalin-containing or alcohol-containing solutions. The complexity and type of microbial testing varies among laboratories. A rapport with the microbiology laboratory should be initiated to facilitate optimal results.

Flow cytometry

Flow cytometry is a laser-based technology, which is able to rapidly count and sort cells based on chemical or physical characteristics. It is often used to diagnose and monitor hematopoietic malignancies through immunophenotyping. Flow cytometry is a process that uses known antibodies directed at surface proteins (antigens) on the cell membrane. Cell viability is imperative, as dead cells can create artifactual or nonspecific antibody binding. Therefore, care must be taken to place the collected cytology specimen in appropriate transport media to maintain viability and arrange for rapid transportation to the laboratory for processing. In properly collected specimens, leukemia or lymphoma subtypes can be differentiated by the unique antibody profile exhibited.[26]

Cell block

A cell block is a useful method to increase the diagnostic accuracy of EUS-FNA, particularly when on-site evaluation is not available. In addition, it is a complementary preparation that can provide confirmatory or additional information alongside the direct smears. The cell block links the cytologic smears to histology by displaying tissue fragments in an architectural pattern. A cell block utilizes the residual aspirate in the needle, small tissue fragments (too dense to smear), material trapped in blood clot, and any excess cellular matter, and allows for it to be histologically evaluated. The composite material collected in fluid is centrifuged, and the pellet is subsequently bonded to form a tissue fragment, then it is embedded in paraffin, sectioned, and stained. Aside from H&E stains, immunohistochemical stains, special stains, and molecular analysis can be performed on the cell block if sufficient material is present.[28] The information obtained from cell-block evaluation and analysis can be instrumental in diagnosis and clinical management.[29,30]

Molecular testing

More recently, the application of molecular analysis has been applied to cytology specimens. Several peer-reviewed publications have used and supported the suitability of cytology specimens for molecular analysis. This utility has best been demonstrated when tissue is acquired in a minimally invasive manner (eg, EUS-FNA), as molecular testing on cytologic specimens has further refined diagnosis, determined prognosis, predicted therapeutic response, and monitored disease relapse/progression.[28,31] With the continuously increasing number of molecular therapeutic options, the demand for molecular testing of small specimens has also increased. Given that small amounts of material can be used for molecular characterization, the endoscopist must be familiar with the criteria for suitability because testing procedures, assay methodologies, and laboratory capabilities vary. For example, one molecular laboratory may require 10 unstained slides with 5-μm thick sections of the tumor tissue collected in cell block, whereas another laboratory may require more or fewer unstained slides or the entire cell block. Therefore, the burden of procuring enough tissue and determining the suitability of the specimen for molecular testing is incumbent on the cooperative effort of the health care team (the referring internist/oncologist, endoscopist, and pathologist).

PREPARATION AND PROCESSING

When placing a slide on a microscope stage for cytologic evaluation, there is an expectation that the slide is satisfactory for rapid assessment. It is presumed that the slide is going to be properly smeared with minimal, if any, crush artifact, showing an appropriately stained monolayer of cells with preserved morphology and clear nuclear detail. Improperly smeared, scant, thick, or poorly preserved slides from sub-optimal preparation make interpretation difficult if not impossible. In many centers, the slides are often prepared by EUS nurses and suite technicians who have been given basic training in slide preparation. However, these personnel do not visualize the specimens microscopically. Therefore, feedback and supervision are essential in ensuring optimal slide preparation.

Glass Slides

There are 3 types of glass microscope slides: plain glass, fully frosted, and frosted single end. The preferred slide is the frosted single end, which provides a frosted (rough) surface for labeling the slide and sufficient space for smearing the aspirate. Slides should be labeled with 2 unique patient identifiers (eg, name, medical record number) to prevent incorrect patient identification. To ensure best laboratory practices, slides should be labeled with the patient's information and site before deposition of the aspirated material. It is good practice to have one staff member responsible for labeling the slides, collection tubes, and requisition forms to minimize the likelihood of error.

Direct Smears

There are varying methods suggested by experts on how to properly deposit aspirated material onto slides. The author typically divides these methods into 2 categories: (1) the snail (stylet) approach and (2) the ape (air-filled syringe) approach.

The snail

Some experts recommend gently expressing a drop of the aspirate onto a slide, in a controlled manner, by using the stylet. Using this approach, the quantity and quality of the cellular material can be appreciated and dispersed among several slides. This method tends to create better smears with minimal (thick tissue or clot) artifact. However, a concern of using this slower controlled method is that if there is scant material it may not be expressed, or a clot may form in the needle that prevents the stylet from advancing.

The ape

The other method commonly used is forcefully expelling the aspirated material onto the slide. This method allows the operator minimal control of specimen deposition, often resulting in splattering of the aspirated material and contamination of the work space, and necessitating additional passes for needle rinsing for ancillary testing (cell block). However, this method is very useful when dealing with sclerotic, fibrotic lesions with solid tissue fragments that must be forcefully expelled, or with thick, viscous, mucinous lesions that adhere to the needle.

Sometimes both methods need to be used, whereby one pass may yield copious fluidic material that should be expelled in a controlled (snail-paced) manner. On the next pass the stylet will not advance, and an air-filled syringe should be pushed into the needle with "gorilla strength" to expel the tissue fragment onto the slide.

Direct Smear Technique

1. Once the slide is labeled appropriately, place the beveled edge of the needle onto the glass slide near the frosted (labeled) end. A smearing slide can be placed at a 45° angle to minimize splatter (**Fig. 2**).
2. Express the aspirated material using the stylet, only allowing one drop of material to be placed on the slide. If excess material is expressed, see Handling Bloody or Excessive Specimens.

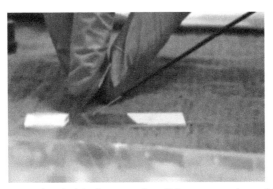

Fig. 2. The endosonographer holds the smearing slide at an angle and the beveled edge down to prevent splatter, contamination of the area, and loss of the aspirated material.

3. Place additional drops of material onto slides as needed; a minimum of 2 slides per pass is recommended (**Fig. 3**).
4. A second slide will be used as a spreader slide to make the smear. The spreader slide is placed firmly over the droplet in a perpendicular direction, which will cause the droplet to spread out slightly by capillary action.
5. While firmly holding the spreader slide down, gently pull it in a downward motion along the length of the slide. Do not attempt to separate the slides during the smearing process (**Fig. 4**).
6. Repeat steps 4 and 5 on the additional slides that contain droplets.
7. Any additional material can be placed in collection fluid (medium or fixative) for further analysis.

Materials for Ancillary Testing

Carrying solutions

When the cellular aspirate containing tissue fragments and cell groups is isolated from the body, a sequence of changes is initiated. Bacteria begin to colonize, flourish, and consume the tissue, while enzymatic activity leads to autolysis or programmed cell death. Therefore, it is imperative to halt these processes by immediate placement of the smears or rinsed material into a fixative or physiologic solution.

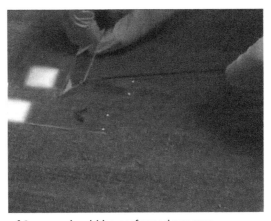

Fig. 3. A minimum of 2 passes should be performed per pass.

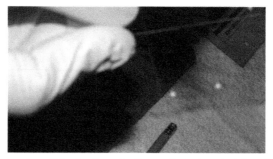

Fig. 4. Press the smearing slide firmly onto the aspirated material and slide in one fluid motion.

Fixatives are solutions that rapidly penetrate the cell to prevent the morphologic and chemical degradation of the aspirated material. By halting the enzymatic activity that occurs through normal cell death (autolysis), the fixative kills the cells in such a way that not only maintain structural integrity but also enhances the cells' sturdiness, thus changing the cellular material to insoluble contents. These changes protect the tissue fragments and cells from distortion during histologic processing (dehydration, embedding, and sectioning). Fixation also allows for better visibility of the air-dried (Diff-Quik) and wet-fixed (Papanicolaou) stains. Furthermore, fixatives prevent the growth of organisms that could possibly consume the cell groups or tissue fragments.

Fixatives are cytotoxic, and care must be taken when using these solutions. Common fixatives used in EUS-FNA are 95% ethyl alcohol, neutral buffered formalin (10% formaldehyde in phosphate-buffered saline), CytoRich Red, CytoLyt, and numerous spray fixatives (SprayFix, Aerocell, and so forth). Spray fixatives are an alternative to liquid (alcohol) fixation, and may be desirable for some centers as they eliminate the need for fixative containers and allow for easy transport. Many of these fixatives dissolve mucus, lyse red blood cells, and reduce protein precipitation, allowing for better visibility and isolation of the diagnostic material. Regardless of the type of fixative or technique (wet or spray fixation) used, if performed correctly, cytologic details should be visualized with minimal artifact.

Physiologic solutions typically used in EUS-FNA are fluids composed of salts and sugars intended to act as cell media for maintaining the aspirated tissue. The purpose of using these solutions is to maintain fluid homeostasis and preserve cellular integrity without killing the cells. Sometimes it is advantageous or necessary to rinse the entire specimen into physiologic solution because viable tissue is required for further analyses (ie, cultures, flow cytometric evaluation, and molecular genetics analysis). These solutions create an isotonic "natural" environment for the cellular aspirate, while maintaining the pH of the solution through buffers. There are numerous physiologic solutions available that contain varying components to make them more tissue specific. For example, RPMI 1640 is a cell-culture medium that has a high phosphate level and is very effective at cultivating and maintaining human lymphoid cells. It is often the carrying solution of choice for specimens being evaluated for lymphoma by flow-cytometric analysis. Typically in EUS-FNA, normal saline, Hanks balanced salt solution, and RPMI 1640 are used as physiologic solutions.

The endosonographer must now be aware that physiologic solutions (cell media) will only temporarily maintain specimen stability, despite the additives that may be present in the carrying solution. Rapid loss of viability over a 24-hour period has been noted with some of these solutions. Moreover, depending on the metabolic activity of the cellular aspirate, the nutrients may be consumed relatively quickly, and the degradation process will ensue regardless of the physiologic agent used. If the physiologic solution containing the aspirate is going to be delayed in transportation to the laboratory, refrigeration is suggested to slow the metabolic activity of the cell and to maintain cell integrity and diagnostic yield. In addition to maintaining the integrity of the cellular aspirate and processing possibilities, the endoscopist must recognize that the choice of fixative or medium needs to be congruent with the laboratory's preferences, as the risk to laboratory personnel must be considered when placing certain (infectious) samples into physiologic solutions.

ASSESSMENT

For optimal assessment of the EUS fine-needle aspirate, it is suggested that a cytopathologist or cytotechnologists be present in the EUS suite during the procedure. A recent meta-analysis used meta-regression to show that the presence of on-site cytopathology was the only significant variable in the diagnostic accuracy of EUS-FNA of pancreatic adenocarcinoma.[8] This finding is not surprising, as several studies have shown that on-site evaluation reduces the rate of nondiagnostic samples, and the absence contributes to sampling error and low diagnostic yield. In addition, on-site assessment reduces the number of passes needed to obtain a diagnosis, thereby reducing the risk of procedure-related complications.[12,32,33]

Although ideal, on-site cytopathology assistance may not be available for a multitude of reasons, this does not mean that the tissue collected from the EUS-FNA procedure cannot be evaluated by the practitioner for sufficiency. The practitioner must be aware that cytologic assessment is much more than merely looking at cells. Evaluation of cells under the microscope is the end product to a process that begins as the sample is expressed from the needle. It is akin to baking a cake; it requires the right ingredients and correct preparation to turn out correctly. For the independent endosonographer, this includes correct patient identification and proper labeling of slides and specimen containers, proper smearing techniques, proper staining techniques and stains, and, if ambitious, perhaps even a microscope.

The following sections discuss techniques that the independent or semi-independent practitioner can use to better assess diagnostic sufficiency if on-site pathology is not available or readily assessable. The endosonographer may choose to incorporate some, if not all of the suggested techniques mentioned. It is important to bear in mind that even if on-site assessment cannot be provided, the laboratory may be willing to assist the practitioner in setting up a space within or near the EUS suite for smearing and staining, as this may have better cost benefit, increased efficiency, and improved patient care.

Technique/Procedure

Adequacy assessment (quantity and quality of material)

Practitioners of ultrasound-guided FNA often are well aware that it is critical to determine whether there is adequate material present in the sample obtained. This assessment can be difficult even when on-site cytopathology assistance is available, as the cytotechnologist, cytopathology fellow, or pathologist might imply that even though some diagnostic material is present, it may not be sufficient for definitive diagnosis. This situation may occur more frequently if initial or preliminary assessment is performed by one cytopathologist and the subsequent final report is issued by a second pathologist who disagrees with the initial assessment (interobserver variability). The reason for this conundrum is 2-fold: (1) a copious amount of aspirate does not equate to a sufficient amount of diagnostic material; and (2) limited material (even if preliminarily considered to be diagnostic) equates to a limited diagnosis.

Visual inspection of smears

The gross appearance of the FNA sample has been long used by cytopathology personnel as a tool to estimate the cellularity and likelihood of diagnostic material on the smear (**Figs. 5** and **6**). Often, to minimize the procedural time the slide that grossly appears to be more cellular is examined microscopically first, permitting the cytotechnologist or cytopathologist to render the diagnosis more rapidly, thereby reducing the number of passes and allowing for any additional material to be triaged appropriately. However, because laboratory personnel that participate in on-site assessment use microscopes, the value of gross assessment is often not explicitly stated. However, a few publications have examined the predictive value of the gross assessment of smears on the diagnostic accuracy, and suggest that this may be useful for non–cytology-trained practitioners, particularly when on-site evaluation is not readily accessible.[10,11]

Visual inspection of collected fluid

Liquids The gross appearance of the aspirated fluid can vary from blood-tinged to hemorrhagic, mucinous, purulent, or serous. The practitioner can observe characteristics, such as the color (ie, brownish or chocolate-colored, straw-colored, yellowish, whitish, or even clear). In addition, as the material is expressed observations can be made regarding viscosity and consistency (gelatinous, mucoid, turbid, watery, and so forth). The question often posed is, "Is the appearance of this fluid associated with the pathologic nature of lesions?" The answer is often "it may be." There are no visual features of aspirated fluid that are pathognomonic for a particular lesion. For example, the thick yellowish-whitish fluid expressed from the needle may be pus-like inflammation or tumor necrosis in malignant disease. Likewise, copious thick mucinous fluid may be consistent with a mucinous neoplasm or gastroduodenal contaminant. However, the gross appearance can be a useful tool in creating a pathologic differential, especially when taking the clinical history and endosonography imaging findings into consideration. The volume of material collected, in addition to

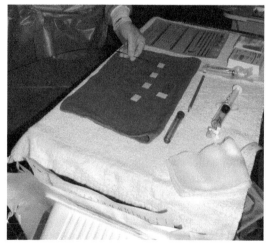

Fig. 5. Visual inspection being performed by the endosonographer to evaluate the quality and quantity of the material expressed from the needle.

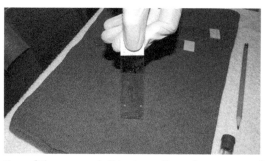

Fig. 6. Gross inspection of the smeared slide shows tissue fragments and granular material.

the color and consistency, also serves as a crude assessment of cellularity (**Fig. 7**). Attempts should be made through an ample number of passes to avoid paucicellular aspirates.

Semisolid aspirate (the worm) Expression of material from larger needles (22- or 19-gauge) can often yield macroscopic "worm-like" matter. These cohesive, semi-solid, slender fragments of tissue can also be informative. Similarly to the liquid aspirate, the worm-like tissue fragment can be grossly assessed. The material can range in consistency from gelatinous and soft to firm and rubbery. Likewise, it can be red or chocolate-brown and hemorrhagic or tan-white, and possibly diagnostic. The appearance of this core-like material can help to gauge if diagnostic material may be present. If the entire tissue piece is red-brown it is most likely blood, whereas if portions of the worm-like tissue are pink or lighter it is not blood. This aspect can be very important when trying to determine whether diagnostic material is present. If there are several pieces of tan-white tissue fragments present floating in the fixative or physiologic solution, there is a greater likelihood that diagnostic material is present. If concerned, a portion of the pink or tan-white tissue can be smeared or touch-prepped (the tissue is gently pressed against the slide) and rapidly stained to see if diagnostic material is present. Tan-white tissue is sometimes firm and rubbery and very difficult to smear, but these dense low-cellularity fragments sometimes consist of desmoplastic or sclerotic tissue.

Options for Handling

Needle rinsing
Needles can be rinsed, after smears and touch-preps have been prepared or as an alternative to direct smears. Various solutions can be used to express any residual

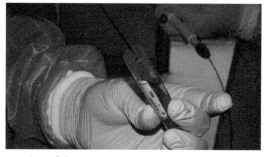

Fig. 7. The visual inspection of the expressed material into the collection medium allows for crude assessment of cellularity.

fluid in the needle, such as normal saline, balanced-salt or electrolyte solution, or culture medium (Cellgro, RPMI 1640). The choice of fluid may depend on the preference of the laboratory and its preferred processing techniques. However, if using fixatives or cytotoxic agents (alcohol, CytoLyt, CytoRich Red, formalin) as a rinse to remove residual cells from the needle, care should be taken to not reintroduce the needle to tissue in vivo. The endosonographer should be aware that the choice of solution for rinsing may restrict the ancillary study choices. This decision is crucial when cytopathology support is not available. Needle rinsing for cell block is a viable alternative for independent practitioners who are uncomfortable or unfamiliar with direct smears and wish to collect diagnostic material without compromising the integrity of the specimen with poorly smeared, fixed, and/or stained slides. There are occasions when no diagnostic material or limited material appears on direct smears, and the washings actually provide or confirm a suspected diagnosis. However, as a rule of thumb, if the direct smears are negative or nondiagnostic, the probability of detecting malignancy from the material obtained through rinsing is low.

Direct smears
The direct smear technique has been previously discussed in the Preparation and Processing section. However, some samples require a higher complexity of smearing technique to avoid preparation pitfalls that may preclude diagnosis. With the advent of larger needles, greater amounts of material are being obtained in one pass, and expressed onto slides. These aspirates have caused frustration in the EUS suite as the preparer feels ill-equipped to deal with an excessively bloody specimen, leaving the practitioner to wonder whether using a larger needle is feasible, or if the additional material is being mishandled. Techniques that can assist practitioners, nurses, techs, or pathologists who wish to perform direct smears of difficult specimens are now described.

Handling bloody or excessive specimens If excessive material is expressed onto the slide diluted by blood, hemorrhagic clot, or fluid, the following smear technique can be applied.

1. Do not attempt to smear this slide. Smearing will lead to loss of tissue, particularly in less experienced hands. Instead examine the slide and see if any solid nonhemorrhagic (tan-pink or yellowish-whitish) fragments are apparent (**Fig. 8**).

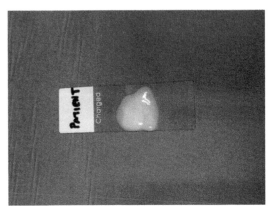

Fig. 8. A slide with copious material present. Smearing of this slide as it appears now would result in loss of sample.

2. Take another (transferring) slide by the frosted end and attempt to pick up one of the nonhemorrhagic fragments using the beveled edge; this is sometimes referred to as the "pick and smear" technique (**Fig. 9**).
3. On a clean properly labeled slide, tap 1 drop of tissue from the beveled edge of the transferring slide. The drop should be placed centrally near the frosted end for adequate room for smearing (**Fig. 10**).
4. Place a smearing slide directly onto the drop of tissue and smear in one fluid motion to the end of the slide (**Fig. 11**).
5. If there is any residual tissue left on the transferring slide, steps 3 and 4 can be repeated. If more smears need to be made, steps 2 to 4 can be repeated.
6. The residual material on the initial slide containing excessive tissue can be scraped into a collection tube for cell-block and/or ancillary testing.

Another method used for handling excessive samples is a touch-preparation technique. This technique can be particularly useful when trying to create direct smears from excessive tissue with core-like material, which may too firm or gelatinous to create a nice monolayer on smearing.

1. Use forceps or the beveled edge of a clean slide to grab the worm-like core or tissue fragment.
2. On a clean properly labeled slide, take the isolated tissue and gently tap it onto the nonfrosted section of the slide in several places. The goal is not to smear the tissue but to allow the superficial cells present in the tissue to adhere to the surface of the slide with each touch.
3. The slide can subsequently be air-dried and rapidly stained, or immediately placed in wet fixative for transport to the laboratory.
4. The residual material on the initial slide containing excessive tissue along with the core-like fragment can be placed into a collection tube for cell-block and/or ancillary testing.

Handling mucoid specimens The mucoid aspirate can be difficult to handle. Mucin is thick, viscous, sticky material that has a gelatinous appearance. Preparing direct

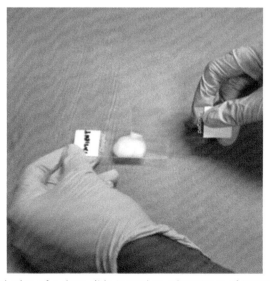

Fig. 9. The beveled edge of a clean slide is used to select tissue of interest.

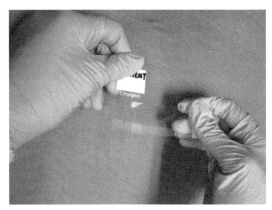

Fig. 10. Gently tap the selected tissue into a clean slide.

smears from these samples can be challenging, as the mucinous material does not dry rapidly and proves difficult in smearing as a monolayer. Moreover, mucoid material can obscure diagnostic tissue fragments on air-dried direct smears and make rapid interpretation difficult. If abundant mucoid material is expelled from the needle, a transferring slide can be used to dilute the material, similarly to handling bloody specimens. Direct smears prepared for Papanicolaou staining should permit visualization of diagnostic material. Some wet-fixed alcohol-based solutions are designed to dissolve mucin to concentrate the cellular material. In addition, for samples collected for specimen processing, mucolytic agents can be used by laboratory personnel if needed.

Postaspiration protocol
On completion of the aspiration of the specimen and triaging of the material for processing, care should be taken to clean the work area and discard all contaminated disposable materials properly. Biologic spills can be cleaned with alcohol, bleach, or other disinfecting agents. It is imperative to clean between cases to avoid cross-contamination.

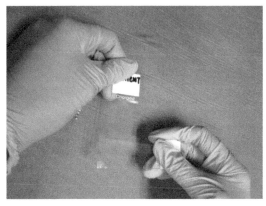

Fig. 11. Smearing of the slide in one smooth motion results in an even distribution of the sample.

On-Site Evaluation

Presence of a cytopathologist

In the author's opinion, the most valuable aspect of on-site assessment is the dialogue generated between the cytopathologist and endosonographer. This rapport facilitates a close working relationship and creates an effective cytopathology-endoscopy team rather than two separate entities working separately to achieve the common goals of diagnostic accuracy and optimal patient management. In doing so, the results are much improved. Not only is on-site assessment and a preliminary diagnosis provided, but a differential diagnosis that will determine whether ancillary testing should be performed will be generated. Moreover, pertinent information, which would have not been included on an ordinary requisition form, may be shared with the pathologist verbally. The information generated through on-site dialogue also may assist in decisions regarding appropriate referrals to specialists so that disease-specific therapeutic interventions can be promptly initiated. In addition, on-site evaluation assists the physician during the procedure, for stage-specific interventions and triaging the aspirate appropriately, to ensure that ancillary studies such as clinical mutational analysis, cultures and PCR for organism, flow cytometry, immunocytochemical analysis, and molecular gene rearrangements are performed as needed. If on-site evaluation is not available and the diagnostic accuracy is lower than expected, expert consultation may be warranted.[34]

Self-assessment

Though seemingly intuitive, the presence of rapid on-site evaluation (ROSE) has been shown to improve patient health management and minimize the likelihood of nondiagnostic specimens and repeat procedures, translating into significant savings in health care dollars. However, despite the advantages, this practice model is not available at many centers because of time-efficiency and cost optimization. Although studies have been published showing that the pathologist is better than the cytotechnologist or endoscopist at on-site evaluation, the literature supports the value of diagnostic adequacy even if only through gross assessment. Therefore it is not surprising that many advanced training programs are providing EUS fellows with procedure-focused cytopathology training, and formal cytopathology workshops and mini-clerkships to practicing endosonographers who perform EUS-FNA. In no way does this substitute for ROSE by a cytopathologist, but it helps in distinguishing nondiagnostic from diagnostic specimens and may assist the independent practitioner in triaging the specimen for ancillary studies.[35] Along these lines, the next 2 sections show common microscopic findings from direct smear (air-dried) preparation in EUS-FNA.

Benign and normal findings An integrated approach that combines imaging studies, clinical presentation, and patient history is recommended when performing cytomorphologic evaluation. Knowing the clinical context will assist in making the most appropriate assessment of the stained smears. This section covers the common normal or benign cellular components visualized on EUS-FNA cytology.

Benign duodenal epithelial cells Fragments of benign duodenal epithelium can be aspirated during transduodenal FNA of pancreatic lesions. Normal duodenal epithelial mucosa typically appears in large cohesive clusters. Cytomorphologically, in tissue fragments the epithelial groups can display prominent papillary finger-like projections. One of the key features to help distinguish duodenal "contaminant" from pancreatic mucosa is the presence of goblet cells. Within duodenal mucosal clusters, there are scattered cells with large intracytoplasmic vacuoles and eccentrically located nuclei;

these represent goblet cells. Microscopically, on low power, goblet cells can appear as white clear spaces in the duodenal epithelium; benign pancreatic epithelium does not have goblet cells (**Fig. 12**).

Benign gastric epithelium Ordinarily benign gastric epithelial cells are arranged in orderly cohesive sheets. The epithelial cells are small and uniform. It can be difficult to distinguish gastric mucosal cells from low-grade mucinous cystic neoplastic epithelium on direct smear preparation, and this can be a diagnostic pitfall. Clinical correlation must be exercised to help distinguish these 2 cell types (**Fig. 13**).

Benign pancreatic acini Normal pancreatic acinar cells are small and have granular cytoplasm. Unlike benign pancreatic ductal cells that are arranged in a honeycomb pattern, acinar cells are arranged in an acinar pattern, meaning that the nuclei are peripherally located and that the centers of the round, grape-like clusters are devoid of cells (**Fig. 14**). The normal pancreas is predominantly composed of acinar cells.

Benign pancreatic ductal cells Normal pancreatic ductal cells form organized monolayer sheets. The nuclei are small, round, evenly spaced, and uniform, giving the appearance of a honeycomb arrangement in cluster (**Fig. 15**).

Chronic pancreatitis Chronic pancreatitis can display various cytomorphologic appearances including dense fragments of fibrous tissue with low cellularity admixed with drunken honeycombs, and scattered benign pancreatic acinar cells and ductal sheets with lymphoplasmacytic infiltrates (**Fig. 16**).

Reactive lymph node The reactive lymphoid aspirate has an array of lymphocytes, ranging from small mature lymphocytes to large activated lymphocytes with open chromatin. Mitotic activity can be seen. Tingible body macrophages and a range of maturation are characteristic of reactive hyperplasia (**Fig. 17**).

Benign squamous epithelium Squamous cells may be present as contaminants from the oral mucosa or esophagus. Superficial and intermediate squamous cells have abundant dense cytoplasm with low nucleus-cytoplasm (N/C) ratios (**Fig. 18**).

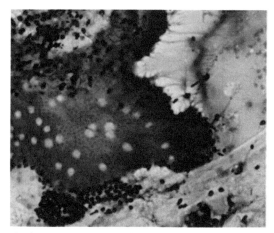

Fig. 12. Gastrointestinal contaminant. Duodenal epithelium with goblet cells appearing as clear white spaces, creating a "starry sky" appearance. Wispy mucin is present in the background (pancreas FNA, direct smear, Diff-Quik; original magnification ×100).

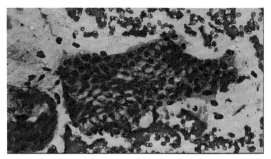

Fig. 13. Gastric contaminant. Gastric foveolar epithelium with back-to-back clear white spaces, similar to bubble wrap (pancreas FNA, direct smear, Diff-Quik; original magnification ×400).

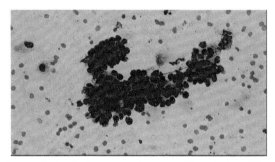

Fig. 14. Benign acinar cells typically appear in grape-like clusters. The nucleus is usually round and peripherally located, with granular cytoplasm (pancreas FNA, direct smear, Diff-Quik; original magnification ×400).

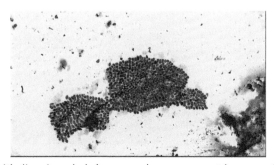

Fig. 15. Ductal epithelium in orderly honeycomb arrangement (pancreas FNA, direct smear, Diff-Quik; original magnification ×100).

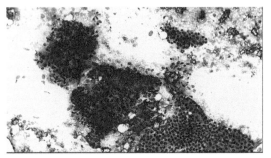

Fig. 16. Chronic pancreatitis. Stromal fibrous and ductal epithelium with mild nuclear atypia and crowding. A cluster of acinar cells is seen in the right upper field (pancreas FNA, direct smear, Diff-Quik; original magnification ×100).

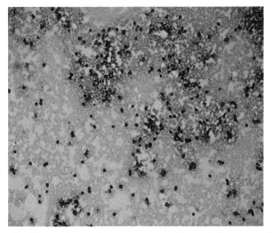

Fig. 17. Reactive node. The aspirate shows a range of lymphoid maturation. Small mature lymphocytes are admixed with slightly larger and very large lymphocytes. A mitotic nucleus can be seen (lymph node, direct smear, Diff-Quik; original magnification ×40).

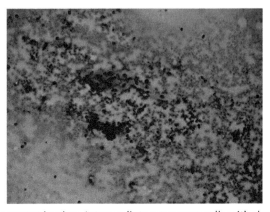

Fig. 18. Squamous contamination. Intermediate squamous cells with dense cytoplasm and round nuclei. Scattered mature lymphocytes are present in the background (lymph node, direct smear, Diff-Quik; original magnification ×40).

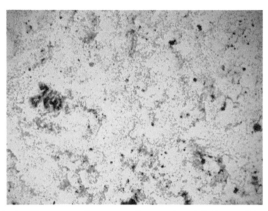

Fig. 19. Degenerated cells, macrophages, and granular debris consistent with pseudocyst contents (pancreas FNA, direct smear, Diff-Quik; original magnification ×40).

Pseudocyst EUS-FNA of pseudocysts typically yields cloudy and turbid fluid. The aspirate is composed primarily of inflammatory cells, macrophages, and granular debris (**Fig. 19**).

Acute inflammation of bile duct Bile-duct strictures may be the result of benign inflammation or malignancy. The normal honeycomb epithelium may be replaced by ductal epithelium with nuclear overlapping, increased N/C ratio, and nuclear irregularity. The presence of numerous inflammatory cells should caution against the diagnosis of malignancy (**Fig. 20**).

Common lesions
Non-Hodgkin B-cell lymphoma Atypical lymphoid populations should behoove the endoscopist to collect specimen for flow cytometry, particularly if there is diffuse lymphadenopathy. The atypical cells are typically intermediate to large in size, with open chromatin and conspicuous nucleoli. A monotonous population can sometimes be visualized (**Fig. 21**).

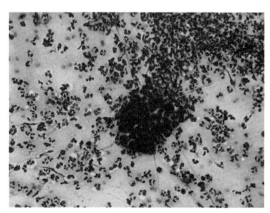

Fig. 20. Ductal epithelium can display marked atypia in an inflammatory milieu. This patient had a recent stent placement. No malignancy was identified (bile duct, direct smear, Diff-Quik; original magnification ×200).

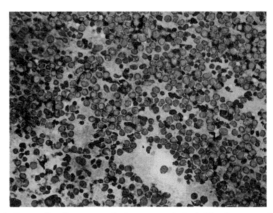

Fig. 21. Two populations of cells can easily be appreciated. The larger cells are monotonous in appearance. Subsequent flow-cytometric analysis demonstrated a monoclonal B-cell lymphoma (lymph node, direct smear, Diff-Quik; original magnification ×200).

Intraductal papillary mucinous neoplasm The epithelial sheets and clusters in intraductal papillary mucinous neoplasm often show slightly disorganized papillary fragments. The tumor cells have irregular nuclear contours and contain cytoplasmic vacuoles. A mucinous background is typical (**Fig. 22**). Sampling may not be representative of the degree of dysplasia, as an invasive component may be present.

Serous cystadenoma The aspirates are often paucicellular and can sometimes be misdiagnosed as "nondiagnostic." Rarely, an aspirate shows a few groups of mono-layered bland epithelial cells with round nuclei (**Fig. 23**).

Pancreatic endocrine neoplasm The aspirate can show neoplastic cells singly and/or in dyshesive groups. The neoplastic cells can have a monotonous appearance (**Fig. 24**), eccentrically located oval nuclei (**Fig. 25**), and septate vacuoles (**Fig. 26**).

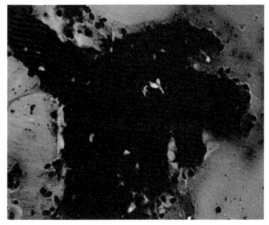

Fig. 22. Ductal epithelium in a papillary arrangement with nuclear atypia, intracytoplasmic vacuoles, and abundant mucin in the background consistent with intraductal papillary mucinous neoplasm (pancreas FNA, direct smear, Diff-Quik; original magnification ×200).

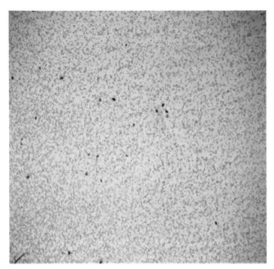

Fig. 23. Paucicellular sample with scattered histiocytes are typical of a serous cystadenoma (pancreas FNA, direct smear, Diff-Quik; original magnification ×40).

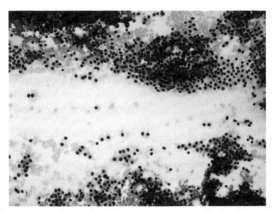

Fig. 24. Neuroendocrine neoplasm showing monotonous cells singly and in groups. The cells characteristically have uniform rounded nuclei and abundant cytoplasm (pancreas FNA, direct smear, Diff-Quik; original magnification ×40).

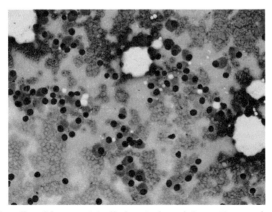

Fig. 25. Neoplastic cells with eccentrically located nuclei creating a plasmacytoid appearance (pancreas FNA, direct smear, Diff-Quik; original magnification ×400).

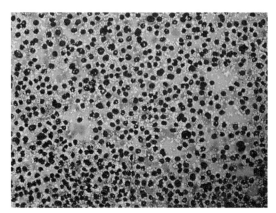

Fig. 26. Neuroendocrine neoplasm with a distinct bubbly appearance caused by numerous intracytoplasmic vacuoles. Endocrine atypia can also be appreciated (pancreas FNA, direct smear, Diff-Quik; original magnification ×200).

Solid pseudopapillary tumor The EUS aspirate shows uniform neoplastic epithelioid cells. If tissue fragments are procured, the neoplastic cells may be found clinging to branching fibrovascular cores as well as being dispersed singly (**Fig. 27**).

Signet-ring carcinoma The aspirate characteristically shows single and small clusters of relatively uniform epithelial cells with intracytoplasmic mucin; the nucleus is often eccentrically displaced, creating the signet-ring appearance (**Fig. 28**).

Ductal adenocarcinoma The EUS aspirate may show single and clusters of malignant epithelial cells with pleomorphism, nuclear crowding, hyperchromasia, irregularity, and overlapping. Huge pleomorphic malignant cells can easily be distinguished from benign honeycomb epithelium (**Fig. 29**). Desmoplastic fibrotic stroma may be a significant component (**Fig. 30**). The aspirate can be hemorrhagic, inflammatory, or necrotic (**Figs. 31** and **32**), and a malignant mucinous component may also be present (**Fig. 33**).

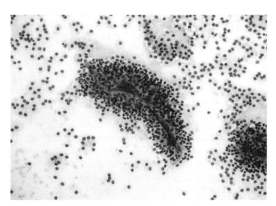

Fig. 27. The tumor cells are small, uniform, and relatively monotonous. A branching capillary surrounded by these bland cells are suggestive of a solid pseudopapillary neoplasm (pancreas FNA, direct smear, Diff-Quik; original magnification ×100).

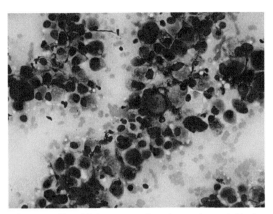

Fig. 28. Loosely discohesive cells with intracytoplasmic mucin and displaced nuclei (stomach, direct smear, Diff-Quik; original magnification ×400).

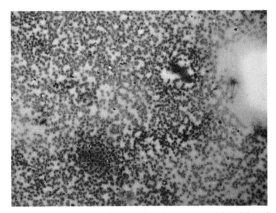

Fig. 29. Large malignancies can have hemorrhagic centers. This bloody aspirate shows 2 monstrous malignant cells (*right upper*) and a ductal sheet with mild atypia (pancreas FNA, direct smear, Diff-Quik; original magnification ×40).

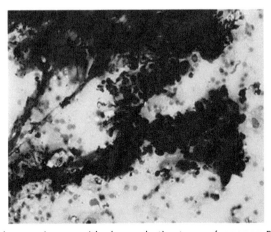

Fig. 30. Ductal adenocarcinoma with desmoplastic stroma (pancreas FNA, direct smear, Diff-Quik; original magnification ×200).

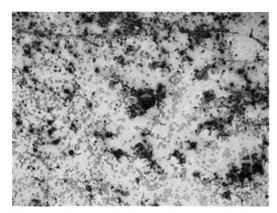

Fig. 31. Rare large bizarre malignant cells in an inflammatory background (pancreas FNA, direct smear, Diff-Quik; original magnification ×40).

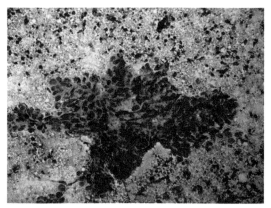

Fig. 32. A malignant sheet of cells in a granular necrotic milieu (pancreas FNA, direct smear, Diff-Quik; original magnification ×200).

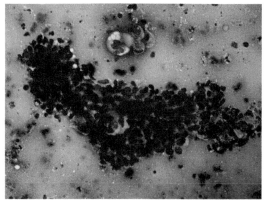

Fig. 33. An overtly malignant ductal sheet with mucinous change (pancreas FNA, direct smear, Diff-Quik; original magnification ×200).

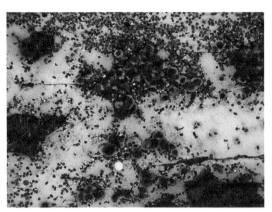

Fig. 34. A lymph node aspirate showing cohesive, haphazardly arranged cells with mucin production. These metastatic malignant cells are easily distinguished from the surrounding lymphocytes (lymph node, direct smear, Diff-Quik; original magnification ×40).

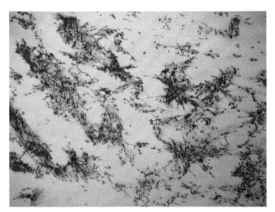

Fig. 35. Numerous spindle cells in a metachromatic matrix consistent with a gastrointestinal stromal tumor (stomach, direct smear, Diff-Quik; original magnification ×40).

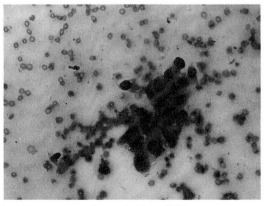

Fig. 36. Large, dark, pleomorphic cells easily identifiable as carcinoma. This tumor was a cholangiocarcinoma (bile duct, direct smear, Diff-Quik; original magnification ×200).

Metastatic carcinoma Metastatic spread to the lymph node is common. Epithelial cells tend to aggregate in cohesive sheets. Caution should be exercised to distinguish from macrophages. Palisading and mucinous change can be present (**Fig. 34**).

Gastrointestinal stromal tumor The cellular aspirate consists of numerous cells with plump spindle to ovoid nuclei embedded in a loose metachromatic stroma (**Fig. 35**). Naked nuclei are often present in the background.

Bile-duct adenocarcinoma Reactive bile-duct atypia can be a diagnostic pitfall; malignancy should be overtly present (**Fig. 36**).

SUMMARY

This article reviews in detail the process of specimen handling and assessment. In addition, for centers that do not have access to on-site cytopathology, practical tips are provided for independent endosonographers to evaluate the specimens independently for diagnostic sufficiency. Having a basic knowledge of cytopathology is imperative for endosonographers who attempt to achieve a greater than 95% diagnostic accuracy from their tissue-acquisition procedures.

REFERENCES

1. Wiersema MJ, Hawes RH, Tao LC, et al. Endoscopic ultrasonography as an adjunct to fine needle aspiration cytology of the upper and lower gastrointestinal tract. Gastrointest Endosc 1992;38(1):35–9.
2. Vilmann P, Jacobsen GK, Henriksen FW, et al. Endoscopic ultrasonography with guided fine needle aspiration in pancreatic disease. Gastrointest Endosc 1992; 38:172–3.
3. Chang KJ, Nguyen P, Erickson R. The clinical utility of endoscopic ultrasound-guided fine-needle aspiration in the diagnosis and staging of pancreatic carcinoma. Gastrointest Endosc 1997;45:387–93.
4. Chhieng DC, Jhala D, Jhala N, et al. Endoscopic ultrasound-guided fine-needle aspiration biopsy: a study of 103 cases. Cancer 2002;96:232–9.
5. Eloubeidi MA, Jhala D, Chhieng DC, et al. Yield of endoscopic ultrasound–guided fine-needle aspiration biopsy in patients with suspected pancreatic carcinoma. Cancer 2003;99:285–92.
6. Eltoum IA, Chhieng DC, Jhala D, et al. Cumulative sum procedure in evaluation of EUS guided FNA cytology: the learning curve and diagnostic performance beyond sensitivity and specificity. Cytopathology 2007;18(3):143–50.
7. Eloubeidi MA, Tamhane A. EUS-guided FNA of solid pancreatic masses: a learning curve with 300 consecutive procedures. Gastrointest Endosc 2005; 61(6):700–8.
8. Hébert-Magee S, Bae S, Varadarajulu S, et al. The presence of a cytopathologist increases the diagnostic accuracy of endoscopic ultrasound-guided fine needle aspiration cytology for pancreatic adenocarcinoma: a meta-analysis. Cytopathology 2013;24(3):159–71.
9. Schmidt RL, Witt BL, Matynia AP, et al. Rapid on-site evaluation increases endoscopic ultrasound-guided fine-needle aspiration adequacy for pancreatic lesions. Dig Dis Sci 2013;58(3):872–82.
10. Nguyen YP, Maple JT, Zhang Q, et al. Reliability of gross visual assessment of specimen adequacy during EUS-guided FNA of pancreatic masses. Gastrointest Endosc 2009;69:1264–70.

11. Mayall F, Cormack A, Slater S, et al. The utility of assessing the gross appearances of FNA specimens. Cytopathology 2010;21:395–7.

12. Alsohaibani F, Girgis S, Sandha GS. Does onsite cytotechnology evaluation improve the accuracy of endoscopic ultrasound-guided fine-needle aspiration biopsy? Can J Gastroenterol 2009;23:26–30.

13. Savoy AD, Raimondo M, Woodward TA, et al. Can endosonographers evaluate on-site cytologic adequacy? A comparison with cytotechnologists. Gastrointest Endosc 2007;65:953–7.

14. Koss LG. Diagnostic cytopathology and its histopathologic bases. 5th edition. Philadelphia: J.B. Lippincott Co; 1992. p. 1570–630.

15. Yang GC, Alvarez II. Ultrafast Papanicolaou stain. An alternative preparation for fine needle aspiration cytology. Acta Cytol 1995;39:55–60.

16. Hirschowitz SL, Mandell D, Nieberg RK, et al. The alcohol-fixed Diff-Quik stain. A novel rapid stain for the immediate interpretation of fine needle aspiration specimens. Acta Cytol 1994;38:499–501.

17. Siegel JD, Rhinehart E, Jackson M, et al, The Healthcare Infection Control Practices Advisory Committee (HICPAC). 2007 guideline for isolations precautions: preventing transmission of infectious agents in healthcare settings. Am J Infect Control 2007;35(10 Suppl 2):S65–164.

18. Eloubeidi MA, Jhala D, Chhieng DC, et al. Late asymptomatic pancreatic metastases from renal cell carcinoma: diagnosis by endoscopic ultrasound-guided fine needle aspiration biopsy with immunocytochemical correlation. Dig Dis Sci 2002; 47(8):1839–42.

19. Chang F, Vu C, Chandra A, et al. Endoscopic ultrasound-guided fine needle aspiration cytology of pancreatic neuroendocrine tumours: cytomorphological and immunocytochemical evaluation. Cytopathology 2006;17:10–7.

20. Jani N, Dewitt J, Eloubeidi M, et al. Endoscopic ultrasound-guided fine-needle aspiration for diagnosis of solid pseudopapillary tumors of the pancreas: a multicenter experience. Endoscopy 2008;40(3):200–3.

21. Hébert-Magee S, Garvin D, Ahlawat S, et al. Lymphoepithelial cyst of the pancreas with sebaceous differentiation: cytologic diagnosis by fine-needle aspiration. Diagn Cytopathol 2009;37:937–9.

22. Bang JY, Hébert-Magee S, Varadarajulu S. Diagnosis of bilateral adrenal metastases secondary to malignant melanoma by EUS-guided FNA. Am J Gastroenterol 2011;106:1862–3.

23. Eloubeidi MA, Luz LP, Crowe DR, et al. Bilateral adrenal gland enlargement secondary to histoplasmosis mimicking adrenal metastases: diagnosis with EUS-guided FNA. Diagn Cytopathol 2010;38:357–9.

24. Wildi SM, Judson MA, Fraig M, et al. Is endosonography guided fine needle aspiration (EUS-FNA) for sarcoidosis as good as we think? Thorax 2004;59:794–9.

25. Itaba S, Yoshinaga S, Nakamura K, et al. Endoscopic ultrasound-guided fine-needle aspiration for the diagnosis of peripancreatic tuberculous lymphadenitis. J Gastroenterol 2007;42:83–6.

26. Al-Haddad M, Savabi MS, Sherman S, et al. Role of endoscopic ultrasound-guided fine-needle aspiration with flow cytometry to diagnose lymphoma: a single center experience. J Gastroenterol Hepatol 2009;24:1826–33.

27. Dabbs DJ. Diagnostic immunohistochemistry. Philadelphia: Churchill Livingstone; 2002.

28. Mitas M, Cole DJ, Hoover L, et al. Real-time reverse transcription-PCR detects KS1/4 mRNA in mediastinal lymph nodes from patients with non-small cell lung cancer. Clin Chem 2003;49:312–5.

29. Ceyhan K, Kupana SA, Bektaş M, et al. The diagnostic value of on-site cytopathological evaluation and cell block preparation in fine-needle aspiration cytology of liver masses. Cytopathology 2006;17:267–74.
30. Kopelman Y, Marmor S, Ashkenazi I, et al. Value of EUS-FNA cytological preparations compared with cell block sections in the diagnosis of pancreatic solid tumours. Cytopathology 2011;22:174–8.
31. Al-Haddad M, Dewitt J, Sherman S, et al. Performance characteristics of molecular (DNA) analysis for the diagnosis of mucinous pancreatic cysts. Gastrointest Endosc, in press.
32. Iglesias-Garcia J, Dominguez-Munoz JE, Abdulkader I, et al. Influence of on-site cytopathology evaluation on the diagnostic accuracy of endoscopic ultrasound-guided fine needle aspiration (EUS-FNA) of solid pancreatic masses. Am J Gastroenterol 2011;106(9):1705–10.
33. Erickson RA, Sayage-Rabie L, Beissner RS. Factors predicting the number of EUS-guided fine-needle passes for diagnosis of pancreatic malignancies. Gastrointest Endosc 2000;51(2):184–90.
34. Alsibai KD, Denis B, Bottlaender J, et al. Impact of cytopathologist expert on diagnosis and treatment of pancreatic lesions in current clinical practice. A series of 106 endoscopic ultrasound-guided fine needle aspirations. Cytopathology 2006;17:18–26.
35. Hayashi T, Ishiwatari H, Yoshida M, et al. Rapid on-site evaluation by endosonographer during endoscopic ultrasound-guided fine needle aspiration for pancreatic solid masses. J Gastroenterol Hepatol 2013;28:656–63.

Endoscopic Ultrasound-Guided Fine-Needle Aspiration Needles
Which One and in What Situation?

Zeid Karadsheh, MD[a], Mohammad Al-Haddad, MD, MSc[b],*

KEYWORDS

- Endoscopic ultrasound • Fine-needle aspiration • EUS sampling techniques
- Cytologic diagnosis

KEY POINTS

- Two decades of experience with EUS-FNA demonstrated high diagnostic accuracy and safety of this procedure.
- Size of the needle, among other factors, can influence the outcome of EUS-FNA.
- Aspiration needles are widely available in 19-gauge, 22-gauge and 25-gauge sizes.
- Location of the lesion to be sampled can influence the choice of needle size.
- 25-gauge needles have been associated with high technical success rates in sampling lesions using the transduodenal approach.
- Histological samples (core biopsies) are required to diagnose certain tumors and are best obtained using 19-gauge needles.

 Videos of the fanning technique and the uncinate process accompany this article

INTRODUCTION

Since its introduction, endoscopic ultrasound (EUS) has been increasingly used for the diagnosis and management of a variety of gastrointestinal (GI) and extraintestinal disorders.[1–4] Due to its minimally invasive nature and the low morbidity associated with it, EUS-guided fine needle aspiration (EUS-FNA) became the technique of choice for sampling lesions within or in close proximity to the GI tract,[5,6] with a high

Conflict of Interest: Dr Al-Haddad has received speaking honoraria from Boston Scientific, Natick, MA.
Funding: None.
[a] Department of Internal Medicine, Brockton Hospital, 680 Centre Street, Brockton, MA 02302, USA; [b] Division of Gastroenterology and Hepatology, Indiana University School of Medicine, 550 North University Boulevard, UH 4100, Indianapolis, IN 46202, USA
* Corresponding author.
E-mail address: moalhadd@iu.edu

diagnostic accuracy exceeding 80% in malignant and benign lesions according to most studies.[7–15]

Several factors influence the diagnostic yield of EUS-FNA, including the experience of the endosonographer, the availability of onsite cytopathology review, the method of cytopathology preparation, the location and physical characteristics of the lesion, and the size of the needle.[16–20] Refinements made to sampling techniques and devices have been the focus of several studies published in the last decade, such as needle size, use of suction during FNA, method of sample expression and processing, and the presence of stylet during puncture.[21–23] Among all these factors, needle size continues to receive the most attention as an independent factor that could increase the diagnostic yield of EUS-FNA.

The most commonly used commercially available EUS-FNA needle sizes are 19, 22, and 25 gauge (G). Choosing a particular size depends on factors such as the type and site of the lesion to be sampled, whether the lesion is solid or cystic, and whether a transgastric or transduodenal approach is required. Needle size also is also determined by whether a cytologic or histologic sample is required, which in turn depends on the nature of the lesion sampled. Smaller needles provide better accessibility due to flexibility in locations where the tip of the scope is angulated and, therefore, are preferred when transduodenal sampling of the pancreatic head or uncinate process is desired.[24,25]

Traditionally, 22-G needles have been the most commonly used and are considered the "default" needles by many endosonographers.[2] A recent change in this trend has been noticeable in many centers, where 25-G needles are increasingly used particularly for transduodenal access.

In the following sections of this review, the authors focus on comparing the different EUS-guided aspiration needles and techniques used to improve the quality of the sample based on the site and type of the lesion to be sampled. The authors critically evaluate needle size as the determinant of diagnostic accuracy as supported by the literature.

Key points

- EUS-FNA is a safe procedure with a high diagnostic accuracy.
- Multiple needle sizes are commercially available including 19, 22, and 25 G.
- The choice of particular needle size depends on multiple factors, including the nature and location of the lesion to be sampled.

SIZE OF NEEDLE

The diagnostic yield of EUS-FNA is directly related to the cytologic quality of the sample. Good sample quality increases the diagnostic accuracy and reduces the need for multiple passes or repeat procedures. To examine the effect of needle size, Lee and colleagues[26] compared the quality of samples obtained by 22-G and 25-G needles in a blinded prospective study. Twelve patients with pancreatic or peripancreatic lesions were enrolled, and each lesion was sampled randomly using 22- and 25-G needles by the same endoscopist. There was no statistically significant difference in the cellular yield of the samples accrued by the 2 needles. However, the endoscopist reported less resistance with the 25-G needle. In a larger study involving the same size needles, Siddiqui and colleagues[27] reported on 131 patients with solid pancreatic masses in a prospective randomized trial. No significant difference in diagnostic yield was observed between 22- and 25-G needles (87.5% vs 95.5%, respectively; $P = .18$). In another study by Fabbri and colleagues,[28] both needles demonstrated 100%

technical success and similar diagnostic accuracy for pancreatic lesions; however, an advantage of the 25-G over the 22-G needle was noted in cytologic diagnosis for malignancy (80% vs 68%). Comparing diagnostic yield from the same lesion sampled consecutively by 22- and 25-G needles, Imazu and colleagues[29] found a trend for numerically higher diagnostic accuracy of the 22-G needle in gastric submucosal tumors compared with the 25-G needle (80% vs 60%), although the difference was not statistically significant. In the same study, a higher diagnostic accuracy was observed in 12 patients with pancreatic masses using the 25-G needle (91.5% vs 75%), although the difference was not statistically significant (**Table 1**). In a large prospective randomized study, Camellini and colleagues[30] compared 22-G with 25-G needles in 127 solid lesions with salvage crossover after 5 inadequate passes or on failure of puncturing the lesion. The number of passes made and specimen adequacy were no different between the 2 groups. More crossover from 22- to 25-G needles was observed in uncinate process masses due to puncture failure. This study suggested a superiority of the 25-G needle in obtaining samples from the pancreatic head. A similar outcome was reported by Sakamoto and colleagues,[31] who reported a higher success rate for reaching a lesion in the uncinate process of the pancreas using the 25-G needle compared with the 22-G needle (see **Table 1**). However, the diagnostic yield for both needles was comparable in technically successful cases.

A meta-analysis by Madhoun and colleagues[32] evaluated 8 studies involving 1292 patients who underwent EUS-FNA with either a 22- or 25-G needle, using surgical histopathology or at least 6 months follow-up as the reference standard for the diagnosis. The sensitivity of the 25-G needle was superior to the 22-G needle (93% vs 85%; $P = .0003$), although their specificity was not different (97% and 100%, respectively).

Fewer studies compared 19-G needle with 22-G and/or 25-G needles. Song and colleagues[25] compared 19-G with 22-G needles for pancreatic and peripancreatic masses in 117 patients. Technical failure occurred in 5 of 60 patients randomized to the 19-G needle, all of which arose in pancreatic head or uncinate process masses and were successfully sampled once crossed over to 22-G needles. Excluding those technical failures, the overall diagnostic accuracy was higher in the 19-G group

Table 1
Technical success rates in sampling pancreatic lesions using 19-, 22-, and 25-G needles as reported in the literature

Study, Year	Needle Size (G)	Number of Patients	Head/Uncinate	Body/Tail	Overall (%)
Imazu et al,[29] 2009	22	12	Not specified	Not specified	75
	25	12	Not specified	Not specified	91.7
Camellini et al,[30] 2011	22	43	Not specified	Not specified	76.6
	25	41	Not specified	Not specified	87.8
Sakamato et al,[31] 2009	19	24	2/12	10/12	50
	22	24	7/12	12/12	79.2
	25	24	12/12	12/12	100
Song et al,[25] 2010	19	60	21/26	34/34	91.7
	22	57	29/29	28/28	100
Fabbri et al,[28] 2011	22	50	42/42	8/8	100
	25	50	42/42	8/8	100

(94.5% vs 78.9%; $P = .015$). Sample quality was also superior in the 19-G needle group ($P = .033$).

Key points

- Most studies showed no difference in quality of a specimen or diagnostic accuracy obtained by different needle sizes once the target lesion was successfully accessed.

- The 25-G needle demonstrated a higher success rate in sampling lesions in the pancreatic head or its uncinate process compared with 22- and 19-G needles.

SAMPLING METHODS AND TECHNICAL FACTORS

FNA technique can affect the quality of samples, and endosonographers vary in the techniques they routinely use to biopsy lesions. Common examples to such variability include the use of suction, performing the fanning technique, and expressing samples using air flushing or by reinserting the stylet. Lee and colleagues[33] compared the quality and diagnostic yield of samples obtained with and without suction in 81 patients with pancreatic masses. Samples expressed by reinserting the stylet and those air flushed were also compared in this study. The number of diagnostic samples, cellularity, and accuracy were higher in the suction group. However, no difference in accuracy, sensitivity, or specificity was found between the stylet versus air-flushed groups, although bloodiness was lower in the air-flushed group. In another trial assessing the effect of suction, 52 solid lesions were randomized to FNA with either suction or no suction. Sensitivity and negative predictive values were higher in the suction group compared with the nonsuction group.[34]

From a practical standpoint, the decision to use suction should also be driven by the nature of the lesion to be sampled. In a vascular target like a lymph node, a nonsuction technique may deliver a better, less bloody sample for the on-site pathologist to render a diagnosis. On the other hand, applying suction in aspirating a fibrotic tumor in the setting of chronic pancreatitis may provide a better result.[35,36]

The fanning technique, in which the trajectory of the needle is altered during FNA using the up/down dial and/or the elevator, was introduced to maximize sampling of various parts of the lesion of interest (Video 1). Bang and colleagues[37] compared this technique with the standard one to sample solid pancreatic masses. The fanning technique was found to be superior, establishing the diagnosis in a fewer number of passes, and resulting in higher first-pass diagnostic rate (85.7% vs 57.7%; $P = .02$). In sampling larger pancreatic masses, this technique provides tissue from the viable peripheral parts of the mass rather than the central part only, which could be necrotic.

The goal of FNA is to provide a confirmatory diagnosis using the least number of passes, which depends largely on the presence of an on-site cytopathologist, who assesses specimen adequacy and provides feedback about the need for further sampling. The optimal number of passes to be performed in the absence of on-site cytopathology services depends on the type of lesion. For example, in solid pancreatic masses, 7 passes have been shown to provide a sensitivity and specificity of 83% and 100%, respectively, whereas in the case of lymph nodes, 5 passes yielded sensitivity and specificity of 77% and 100%, respectively.[38] It is generally recommended that 5 to 7 passes be obtained from pancreatic masses and 3 passes from lymph nodes when an on-site cytopathologist is not available. In this situation, 2 dedicated passes must always be performed and submitted entirely in cell block whenever possible to increase the diagnostic yield, which also allows immunocytochemistry studies (**Fig. 1**).

Key points

- Expression technique may affect the quality of a specimen. Application of suction during FNA followed by air flushing to express the sample seems to provide a better quality specimen, but data remain limited.
- Sampling various parts of the target lesion using the fanning technique has been shown to provide a cytologically superior specimen compared with the standard technique.
- On-site cytopathology offers immediate feedback about the quality of EUS-FNA specimens obtained, and therefore helps improve the diagnostic certainty and minimize the need for repeat procedures.
- It is recommended that 5 to 7 passes be obtained from pancreatic masses and 3 passes from lymph nodes when an on-site cytopathologist is not available.

SITE OF THE LESION

The location of the lesion targeted for sampling affects the choice of needle and the technique to be used. Depending on the site, deep insertion of the echoendoscope, excessive tip angulation, and/or the use of elevator may be necessary. Such maneuvers may increase the resistance to insertion and advancement of the needle. For example, while sampling masses in the head of pancreas or the uncinate process, scope tip angulation is often required to maintain apposition with the mass. This position makes use of larger, stiffer 19-G needles more challenging, and a 22- or 25-G needle is preferred in this case (**Fig. 2**, Video 2). To objectively assess this, Itoi and colleagues[24] evaluated the resistance of various needles during insertion and advancement under several conditions of the endoscope (straight and angulated endoscope position, endoscope tip angulation, and while using the elevator). Less resistance was encountered with the 22- and 25-G needles under almost any position compared with the conventional 19-G needle and 19-G Tru-cut needle.

Location of lesion: practical tips
1. To minimize the overall resistance to needle advancement in the transduodenal approach (regardless of size), it is recommended to place the scope in a short position whenever possible. Although the scope is unstable, the short position facilitates needle exit.
2. Anchoring the scope in the duodenal bulb (long position) is an alternative more stable position; however, more resistance is encountered to advance and withdraw the needle due to the curve in the scope along the greater curvature of the stomach.
3. Air suction also helps bring the wall closer to the probe and further stabilizes the tip of the scope in any position.
4. If the needle cannot be advanced out of the scope because of scope tip deflection, relaxing the big dial straightens the tip of the scope and allows needle advancement into the lesion. Occasionally, it is also necessary to withdraw the scope back into the proximal stomach to achieve this.
5. In the transgastric approach, the use of 19-G needles is facilitated by maintaining a shorter straighter scope. Nevertheless, the thickness of the gastric wall and the wide lumen, which tends to "tent" away during puncture, could increase the difficulty accessing lesions from this location.

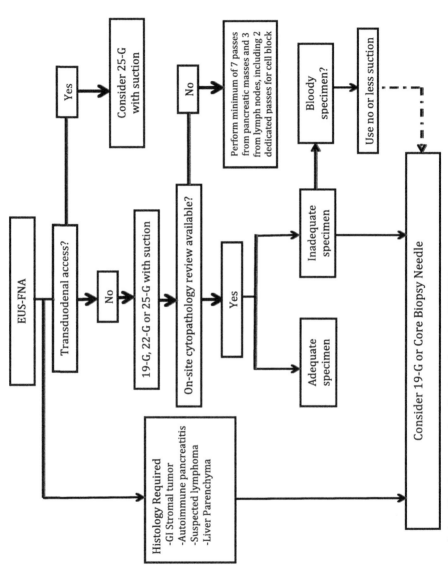

Fig. 1. Proposed general algorithm to approach patients undergoing EUS-FNA.

6. Withdrawing the stylet slightly before puncture exposes the sharp edge of the needle and could facilitate initial puncture.

Key points

- Lesions in the head and uncinate process of the pancreas require transduodenal access, which in turn entails significant endoscope and/or tip angulation. Such lesions can be better accessed with a short scope position and by using smaller needles (22 or 25 G, see **Fig. 1**).

TYPE OF THE SPECIMEN

EUS-FNA is currently the standard procedure for sampling pancreatic masses, and in most cases, cytology alone is adequate to confirm a diagnosis. However, certain conditions such as lymphoma, mesenchymal tumors, and well-differentiated tumors may be difficult to diagnose by cytology alone.[39,40] In addition, the negative predictive value of EUS-FNA does not permit exclusion of malignancy, particularly in the setting of inflammation such as chronic pancreatitis. In the last decade, dedicated fine-needle biopsy (FNB) devices (EUS-FNB) have been developed to acquire larger amount of tissue while preserving the architecture to enable histologic analysis.[41] Such devices include the Quick-Core and more recently released ProCore biopsy needles (Cook Medical, Winston-Salem, NC, USA). These devices were found to provide a correct diagnosis in 96% and 89% of cases, respectively, according to one recent multicenter trial.[42] Further details about such devices will be presented elsewhere in this issue.

Despite the advent of new devices dedicated to the procurement of core biopsies, the classic designation of FNA versus FNB devices has been challenged. A recent prospective study by Bang and colleagues,[43] randomly comparing 22-G FNA to 22-G FNB needles for sampling solid pancreatic masses showed no significant difference in procurement of the core tissue in 56 patients (100% vs 83.3%; $P = .26$) or the presence of diagnostic histologic specimens (66.7% vs 80%; $P = .66$) (**Table 2**).

Rong and colleagues,[44] on the other hand, found that histologic adequacy of the 22-G needle was superior to the 25-G needle in pancreatic masses and submucosal tumors (70.4% vs 61.1%; $P = .33\%$ and 74.1% vs 55.6%; $P = .18$, respectively). However, diagnostic accuracy did not differ between the 2 needles (80.0% vs 78.9%) when

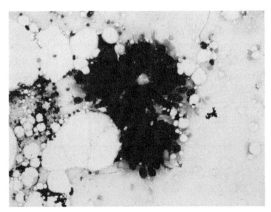

Fig. 2. Cytology smears from the uncinate mass biopsied in Video 1 confirmed adenocarcinoma (Diff-Quick, original magnification ×20).

Table 2
Rate of histologically adequate specimens procured using the 3 common size needles in the literature

Study, Year	Needle Size (G)	Number of Patients	Histologic Adequacy (%)	Location of Biopsy
Iwashita et al,[47] 2012	19	44	43	Pancreas[a]
Yasuda et al,[45] 2006	19	104	98	Lymph nodes
Rong et al,[44] 2012	22	54	70.4	Pancreas
	25	54	61.1	Pancreas
	22	27	74.1	Submucosal tumors
	25	27	55.6	Submucosal tumors
Bang et al,[43] 2012	22, FNA	28	66.7	Pancreas
	22, FNB	28	80	
Larghi et al,[46] 2011	19	120	97.5	Various
Varadarajulu et al,[48] 2012	19[b]	38	94.7	Subepithelial masses Pancreatic (head and uncinate lesions)

[a] Autoimmune pancreatitis cases only included.
[b] A flexible nitinol-based needle was used in all procedures.

both needles were used in the same patient (see **Table 2**). Yasuda and colleagues[45] reported on the accuracy of EUS-FNB for sampling lymphadenopathy with 19-G needles, whereby FNB alone provided an accurate diagnosis of lymphoma in 96% of the patients (see **Table 2**). Eighty-eight percent of the patients (44/50) had sufficient histologic sample to successfully classify their lymphoma according to the World Health Organization classification system. In another study that further demonstrated the adequacy of 19-G needle in providing histologic samples, Larghi and colleagues[46] reported successful histology acquisition in 97% (116/119) of patients enrolled (see **Table 2**). In a rather specific application, the diagnostic accuracy of EUS-FNA using a 19-G needle to obtain a histologic diagnosis of autoimmune pancreatitis was found to be 43% in one study.[47]

Due to the technical challenges associated with accessing lesions through a transduodenal approach, a recently developed flexible needle made of Nitinol became available (Flex 19 G Expect, Boston Scientific, Natick, MA, USA). This device was initially evaluated by Varadarajulu and colleagues[48] in 38 patients, including 32 with pancreatic head or uncinate process lesions. There were no technical failures reported, and histologic samples were adequate in 36 of the 38 patients (93.7%). Similar technical success and tissue yield was reported by another multicenter study published in abstract form that included pancreatic masses among other intramural and extramural lesions (**Figs. 3** and **4**).[49] Despite the limited studies directly comparing the cytologic and histologic yield of EUS acquired samples, larger bore needles such as 19 G are probably better positioned to provide adequate histologic specimens compared with smaller size needles, but further head-to-head comparative studies are needed.

Key points

- Certain lesions or conditions require a histologic specimen in addition to or in lieu of a cytologic one for an accurate diagnosis.
- Dedicated core biopsy needles and 19-G needles should be used to obtain histologic samples when this aids the diagnosis.

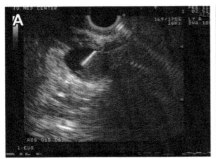
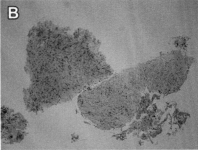

Fig. 3. (*A*) A rectal subepithelial lesion was noted on routine colonoscopy. On EUS, the lesions seemed to originate from the fourth wall layer (muscularis propria) and are partially exophytic. FNB was performed using a 19-G flexible needle. (*B*) Histopathology from the FNB confirmed a gastrointestinal stromal tumor (hematoxylin-eosin, original magnification ×10).

COMPLICATIONS RATE

Complications of EUS-FNA are rare and include bleeding and infection, in addition to pancreatitis in pancreatic biopsies, which collectively occur in about 2% or less of procedures.[50–52] There have been case reports of tumor seeding of the FNA, although this remains rare.[53,54] Appropriate positioning of the tip of the scope, avoiding intervening vessels during puncture, and use of antibiotics when aspirating cystic lesions can help reduce FNA-related complications. Nevertheless, theoretical concerns about FNA-related complications arise, and the size of the needle and the number of passes made may also affect the overall risk of complications. To date, no study has evaluated whether the size of the needle can influence the risk of adverse events. Due to the very low overall rate of EUS-FNA complications, a rather large sample size is needed to demonstrate any potential difference in complications using larger size

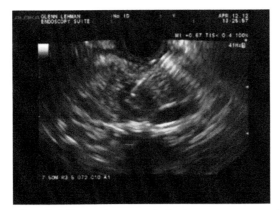

Fig. 4. Multiple small well-delineated pancreatic body masses were noted on computed tomographic imaging in a woman with vague abdominal and weight loss. One of the lesions was sampled using a 19-G needle. Cytology review confirmed metastatic lobular carcinoma of the breast. The patient was treated for this tumor 15 years earlier and was declared to be in remission.

needles. However, it is recommended that the diagnosis be made with the minimal number of passes to avoid unnecessary risks.

Key points

- EUS-FNA is generally a safe procedure with low risk of complications encountered in 2% or less of cases.

SUMMARY

EUS-FNA is a safe procedure with high diagnostic accuracy. Different needles sizes are commercially available including 19, 22, and 25 G. Needle size can potentially influence the diagnostic yield of EUS-FNA and has been evaluated in different studies. In most studies, 25-G needles were clearly superior to 19-G and somewhat the 22-G ones in accessing lesions when the tip of the scope is angulated or when sampling using a long scope position, which are typical scenarios for transduodenal access. Therefore, 25-G needles should be considered first in sampling lesions in the head of the pancreas, in uncinate process or across the second part of the duodenum. Specimen quality was not different among the 3 size needles in most studies. However, larger bore needles seem to be better positioned to provide histologic specimens (core biopsies) once a lesion is accessed. Further head-to-head comparative studies are needed to assess safety and diagnostic yield of the newer core biopsy and the flexible 19-G needles.

SUPPLEMENTARY DATA

Videos related to this article can be found online at http://dx.doi.org/10.1016/j.giec. 2013.08.008.

REFERENCES

1. Vilmann P, Jacobsen GK, Henriksen FW, et al. Endoscopic ultrasonography with guided fine needle aspiration biopsy in pancreatic disease. Gastrointest Endosc 1992;38:172–3.
2. Erikson RA. EUS-guided FNA. Gastrointest Endosc 2004;60:267–79.
3. Mortensen MB, Pless T, Durup J, et al. Clinical impact of endoscopic ultrasound-guided fine needle aspiration biopsy in patients with upper gastrointestinal malignancies. A prospective study. Endoscopy 2001;33:478–83.
4. Shah JN, Ahmad NA, Beilstein MC, et al. Clinical impact of endoscopic ultrasonography on the management of malignancies. Clin Gastroenterol Hepatol 2004;2:1069–73.
5. Gan SI, Rajan E, Adler DG, et al. Role of EUS. Gastrointest Endosc 2007;66: 425–34.
6. Dumonceau JM, Polkowski M, Larghi A, et al. Indications, results, and clinical impact of endoscopic ultrasound (EUS)-guided sampling in gastroenterology: European society of Gastrointestinal Endoscopy (ESGE) Clinical Guideline. Endoscopy 2001;43:897–912.
7. Gress F, Gottlieb K, Sherman S, et al. Endoscopic ultrasonography-guided fine-needle aspiration biopsy of suspected pancreatic cancer. Ann Intern Med 2001; 134:459–64.
8. Suits J, Frazee R, Erickson RS. Endoscopic ultrasound and fine needle aspiration for the evaluation of pancreatic masses. Arch Surg 1999;134:639–43.

9. Chang J, Nguyen P, Erickson RA, et al. The clinical utility of endoscopic ultrasound-guided fine-needle aspiration in the diagnosis and staging of pancreatic carcinoma. Gastrointest Endosc 1997;45:387–93.

10. Bhutani MS, Hawes RH, Baron PL, et al. Endoscopic ultrasound guided fine needle aspiration of malignant pancreatic lesions. Endoscopy 1997;29:854–8.

11. Gress FG, Savides TJ, Sandler A, et al. Endoscopic ultrasonography, fine-needle aspiration biopsy guided by endoscopic ultrasonography, and computed tomography in the preoperative staging of non-small lung cancer: a comparison study. Ann Intern Med 1997;127:604–12.

12. Wiersema MJ, Vazquez-Sequeiros E, Wiersema LM. Evaluation of mediastinal lymphadenopathy with endoscopic US-guided fine-needle aspiration biopsy. Radiology 2001;219:252–7.

13. Fritscher-Ravens A, Sriram PV, Bobrowski C, et al. Mediastinal lymphadenopathy in patients with or without obvious malignancy: EUS-FNA based differential cytodiagnosis in 153 patients. Am J Gastroenterol 2000;95:2278–84.

14. Wallace MB, Silvestri GA, Sahai AV, et al. Endoscopic ultrasound-guided fine needle aspiration for staging patients with carcinoma of the lung. Ann Thorac Surg 2001;72:1861–7.

15. Vazquez-Sequeiros E, Norton ID, Clain JE, et al. Impact of endoscopic ultrasound guided fine-needle aspiration on lymph node staging in patients with esophageal carcinoma. Gastrointest Endosc 2001;53:751–7.

16. Savides TJ. Tricks for improving EUS-FNA accuracy and maximizing cellular yield. Gastrointest Endosc 2009;69:S130–3.

17. Bentz JS, Kochman ML, Faigel DO, et al. Endoscopic ultrasound-guided real-time fine-needle aspiration: clinicopathologic features of 60 patients. Diagn Cytopathol 1998;18:98–109.

18. Mertz MR, Gautam S. The learning curve for EUS-guided FNA of pancreatic cancer. Gastrointest Endosc 2004;59:33–7.

19. Itoi T, Itokawa F, Sofuni A, et al. Puncture of solid pancreatic tumors guided by endoscopic sonography: a pilot study series comparing a Tru-cut and 19-gauge and 22-gauge aspiration needles. Endoscopy 2004;37:362–6.

20. Fritscher-Ravens A, Topalidis T, Bobrowski C, et al. Endoscopic ultrasound-guided fine needle aspiration in focal pancreatic lesions: a prospective intraindividual comparison of two needles assemblies. Endoscopy 2001;33:484–90.

21. Sahai AV, Paquin SC, Gariépy G. A prospective comparison of endoscopic ultrasound-guided fine needle aspiration results obtained in the same lesion, with and without the needle stylet. Endoscopy 2010;42:900–3.

22. Rastogi A, Wani S, Gupta N, et al. A prospective, single-blind, randomized, controlled trial of EUS-guided FNA with and without a stylet. Gastrointest Endosc 2011;74:58–64.

23. Wani S, Gupta N, Gaddam S, et al. A comparative study of endoscopic ultrasound guided fine needle aspiration with and without a stylet. Dig Dis Sci 2011;56:2409–14.

24. Itoi T, Itokawa F, Kurihara T, et al. Experimental endoscopy: objective evaluation of EUS needles. Gastrointest Endosc 2009;69:509–16.

25. Song TJ, Kim JH, Lee SS, et al. The prospective randomized, controlled trial of endoscopic ultrasound-guided fine needle aspiration using 22G and 19G aspiration needles for solid pancreatic and peripancreatic masses. Am J Gastroenterol 2010;105:1739–45.

26. Lee J, Stewart J, Ross W, et al. Blinded prospective comparison of the performance of 22-gauge and 25-gauge needles in endoscopic ultrasound-guided

fine needle aspiration of the pancreatic and peri-pancreatic lesions. Dig Dis Sci 2009;54:2274–81.

27. Siddiqui U, Rossi F, Rosenthal L, et al. EUS-guided FNA of solid pancreatic masses: a prospective randomized trial comparing 22-gauge and 25-gauge needles. Gastrointest Endosc 2009;70:1093–7.

28. Fabbri C, Polifemo AM, Luigiano C, et al. Endoscopic ultrasound-guided fine needle aspiration with 22- and 25-gauge needles in solid pancreatic masses: a prospective comparative study with randomisation of needle sequence. Dig Liver Dis 2011;43:647–52.

29. Imazu H, Uchiyama Y, Kakutani H, et al. A prospective comparison of EUS-guided FNA using 25-gauge and 22-gauge needles. Gastroenterol Res Pract 2009;2009:546390.

30. Camellini L, Carlinfante G, Azzolini F, et al. A randomized clinical trial comparing 22G and 25G needles in endoscopic ultrasound-guided fine-needle aspiration of solid lesions. Endoscopy 2011;43:709–15.

31. Sakamoto H, Kitano M, Komaki T, et al. Prospective comparative study of the EUS guided 25-gauge FNA needle with the 19-gauge Tru-cut needle and 22-gauge FNA needle in patients with solid pancreatic masses. J Gastroenterol Hepatol 2009;24:384–90.

32. Madhoun MF, Wani SB, Rastogi A, et al. The diagnostic accuracy of 22-gauge and 25-gauge needles in endoscopic ultrasound-guided fine needle aspiration of solid pancreatic lesions: a meta-analysis. Endoscopy 2013;45: 86–92.

33. Lee JK, Choi JH, Lee KH, et al. A prospective, comparative trial to optimize sampling techniques in EUS-guided FNA of solid pancreatic masses. Gastrointest Endosc 2013;77:745–51.

34. Puri R, Vilmann P, Saftoiu A, et al. Randomized controlled trial of endoscopic ultrasound-guided fine-needle sampling with or without suction for better cytological diagnosis. Scand J Gastroenterol 2009;44:499–504.

35. Santos JE, Leiman G. Nonaspiration fine needle cytology. Application of a new technique to nodular thyroid disease. Acta Cytol 1988;32:353–6.

36. Kinney TB, Lee MJ, Filomena CA, et al. Fine-needle biopsy: prospective comparison of aspiration versus nonaspiration techniques in the abdomen. Radiology 1993;186:549–52.

37. Bang JY, Magee SH, Ramesh J. Randomized trial comparing fanning with standard technique for endoscopic ultrasound-guided fine-needle aspiration of solid pancreatic mass lesions. Endoscopy 2013;45:445–50.

38. LeBlanc JK, Ciaccia D, Al-Assi MT, et al. Optimal number of EUS-guided fine needle passes needed to obtain a correct diagnosis. Gastrointest Endosc 2004;59:475–81.

39. Erikson RA, Sayage-Rabie L, Beissner S. Factors predicting the number of EUS-guided fine needle passes for diagnosis of pancreatic malignancies. Gastrointest Endosc 2000;51:184–90.

40. Ribeiro A, Vazquez-Sequeiros E, Wiersema LM, et al. Endosonography guided fine needle aspiration biopsy combined with flow cytometry and immunocytochemistry in the diagnosis of lymphoma. Gastrointest Endosc 2001;53:485–91.

41. Levy MJ. Endoscopic ultrasound-guided Trucut biopsy of the pancreas: prospects and problems. Pancreatology 2007;7:163–6.

42. Iglesias-Garcia J, Poley JW, Larghi A, et al. Feasibility and yield of the new EUS histology needle: results from a multicenter, pooled, cohort study. Gastrointest Endosc 2011;73:1189–96.

43. Bang JY, Hebert-Magee S, Trevino J, et al. Randomized trial comparing the 22-gauge aspiration and 22-gauge biopsy needles for EUS-guided sampling of solid pancreatic mass lesions. Gastrointest Endosc 2012;76:321–7.

44. Rong L, Kida M, Yamauchi H, et al. Factors affecting the diagnostic accuracy of endoscopic ultrasonography-guided fine-needle aspiration (EUS-FNA) for upper gastrointestinal submucosal or extraluminal solid mass lesions. Dig Endosc 2012;24:358–63.

45. Yasuda I, Tsurumi H, Omar S, et al. Endoscopic ultrasound-guided fine-needle aspiration biopsy for lymphadenopathy of unknown origin. Endoscopy 2006;38: 919–24.

46. Larghi A, Verna E, Ricci R, et al. EUS-guided fine-needle tissue acquisition by using a 19-gauge needle in a selected patient population: a prospective study. Gastrointest Endosc 2011;74:504–10.

47. Iwashita T, Yasuda I, Doi S, et al. Use of samples from endoscopic ultrasound-guided 10-gauge fine-needle aspiration in diagnosis of autoimmune pancreatitis. Clin Gastroenterol Hepatol 2012;10:316–22.

48. Varadarajulu S, Bang J, Hebert-Magee S. Assessment of the technical performance of the flexible 19-gauge EUS-FNA needle. Gastrointest Endosc 2012; 76:336–43.

49. Al-Haddad M, Ashish A, Aman A. EUS-guided biopsy with a novel 19-gauge fine needle biopsy (FNB) device: multi-center experience. Gastrointest Endosc 2013;77:AB403–4.

50. O'Toole D, Palazzo L, Arotçarena R, et al. Assessment of complications of EUS-guided fine-needle aspiration. Gastrointest Endosc 2001;53:470–4.

51. Adler DG, Jacobson BC, Davila RE, et al. ASGE guideline: complications of EUS. Gastrointest Endosc 2005;61:8–12.

52. Doi S, Yasuda I, Iwashita T, et al. Needle tract implantation on the esophageal wall after EUS-guided FNA of metastatic mediastinal lymphadenopathy. Gastrointest Endosc 2008;67:988–90.

53. Paquin SC, Gariépy G, Lepanto L, et al. A first report of tumor seeding because of EUS-guided FNA of a pancreatic adenocarcinoma. Gastrointest Endosc 2005;61:610–1.

54. Micames C, Jowell PS, White R, et al. Lower frequency of peritoneal carcinomatosis in patients with pancreatic cancer diagnosed by EUS-guided FNA vs. percutaneous FNA. Gastrointest Endosc 2003;58:690–5.

Techniques for EUS-guided FNA Cytology

Sarto C. Paquin, MD, FRCPC, Anand V. Sahai, MD, MSc (EPID), FRCPC*

KEYWORDS

- Endosonography • Fine-needle aspiration • Cytology • Technique • Indications

KEY POINTS

- For solid lesions, the basic endoscopic ultrasound (EUS)-guided fine-needle aspiration (FNA) technique consists of proper positioning and moving of the needle inside the lesion with multiple to and fro movements, under ultrasound guidance.
- Many additions to the basic EUS-FNA technique have been described, but none appear to clearly improve the yield other than moving the needle effectively and in many different areas of the lesion.
- For the goal of obtaining cytologic specimens, there is no clear advantage to use of the stylet, suction, larger diameter needles, or other modified needles.

INTRODUCTION

For the purposes of this article, the authors assume that the goal of solid lesion endoscopic ultrasound (EUS)-guided fine-needle aspiration (FNA) is to obtain material for cytologic smears and/or for a tissue cell block (which can be processed to permit histologic analysis). EUS-guided FNA biopsy (FNAB) differs from FNA in that FNAB refers to sampling techniques designed to obtain a " core" specimen for pure histologic analysis. This article will not address puncture of cystic lesions.

The authors describe a basic EUS-FNA technique that they believe should be used at all times, but that can be modified by changing other variables such as suction or different needle types and sizes.

CYTOLOGY: ADVANTAGES, LIMITATIONS

These issues are beyond the scope of this article and will be addressed by others. Suffice it to say that, in the authors' experience, standard cytology, combined with a cell block (when special stains are required) is largely sufficient to obtain a diagnosis in more than 95% of cases in a standard EUS practice. A true histologic "core" is needed

Centre hospitalier de l'Université de Montréal, 1058 Rue Saint Denis, Montréal, Québec H9E 1A8, Canada
* Corresponding author.
E-mail address: anand.sahai@sympatico.ca

Gastrointest Endoscopy Clin N Am 24 (2014) 71–81
http://dx.doi.org/10.1016/j.giec.2013.08.007
1052-5157/14/$ – see front matter © 2014 Elsevier Inc. All rights reserved.

giendo.theclinics.com

only in cases where tissue structure is important (eg, suspected lymphoma) or in cases where cytologic specimens are often poorly cellular (eg, suspected linitis plastica, leiomyoma, etc.).

INDICATIONS/CONTRAINDICATIONS

Indications for EUS-FNA for tissue acquisition have broadened over time. Tissue sampling is performed most often to confirm suspected cancer,[1] although it may also be useful in benign conditions such as diagnosing sarcoidosis or infections (eg, tuberculosis, fungal disease, etc.). **Box 1** summarizes the common sites for performing EUS-FNA.

Contraindications to EUS-FNA are few. Before performing EUS-FNA, the endosonographer must be certain that there is a reasonable chance that tissue sampling will be clinically useful.

As a general rule, FNA should be avoided in patients with significant coagulopathy (INR>1.2, platelets <100,000, recent use of thienopyridines [eg, clopidogrel], etc.).[2,3] However, the use of aspirin or nonsteroidal antiinflammatory drugs (NSAIDs) is not a problem. Patients receiving anticoagulant therapy such as warfarin or dabigatran should discontinue their medication before the procedure (3–5 days for warfarin, 48 hours for dabigatran). If the patient is at high risk for thromboembolic events, bridge therapy with low molecular weight heparin should be considered. Patients receiving antiplatelet therapy such as (eg, clopidogrel) should also withhold them for 7 to 10 days before the procedure if they carry a low thromboembolic risk.

Some high-risk patients may not safely discontinue their treatment. In these situations, where the risk of stopping anticoagulation is potentially greater than the risk of FNA-induced bleeding (eg, FNA of a large mediastinal node in a patient anticoagulated for massive pulmonary embolus), it may be reasonable to attempt EUS-FNA without stopping anticoagulants, while using a small gauge (25g) needle and minimizing the number of passes (eg, with onsite cytology).

Box 1
Common sites for performing EUS-FNA

Pancreas

Bile duct

Digestive wall lesions[a]

  Suspicious wall thickening

  Subepithelial lesions

Adrenal glands

Liver

Retroperitoneal masses

Lymph nodes

Posterior mediastinum

  Suspicious lymph nodes

  Pulmonary masses[b]

[a] Digestive wall lesions include the esophagus, stomach, duodenum, and rectum.

[b] Pulmonary masses must abut the posterior mediastinum to be vizualized under EUS.

Finally, certain anatomic challenges may also contraindicate EUS-FNA, such as a large vessel or duct interposing itself between the targeted lesion and the ultrasound probe. Lymph nodes may not be accessible if the primary mass is preventing direct node sampling, carrying the risk of false-positive results. **Box 2** provides an overview to EUS-FNA contraindications.

THE BASIC EUS-FNA TECHNIQUE

For didactic purposes, the basic EUS-FNA technique has been broken down into multiple components. In reality, the process should be a smooth, seamless process.

Identify and Characterize the Lesion

Obviously, the lesion must be identifiable before FNA can be attempted. However, the initial assessment should also try to characterize the lesion as solid or cystic because the indications and risks of puncture of cystic lesions are not the same as for solid lesions. The technique of EUS-FNA for cystic lesions is beyond the scope of this article.

Assess the Indication and Rule out Contraindications for EUS-FNA

Not all solid lesions should undergo FNA. FNA should be performed only if the benefits outweigh the risks. Since the risks of solid lesion EUS-FNA are generally small, it is probably reasonable to perform EUS-FNA in most indeterminate solid lesions, but there are notable exceptions. If there is any doubt, this issue should be addressed with the referring physician before the procedure (or even during the procedure), if necessary.

EUS-FNA should be avoided if it clearly does not influence management or treatment, if there is a risk of tumor seeding that could worsen clinical outcomes, if there is an excessive risk of puncture-related complications (eg, bleeding, infection, trauma to surrounding structures, hypertensive crisis [eg, possible pheochromocytoma]).

When faced with the possibility of performing FNA on multiple sites, one should focus on the lesion likely to provide the most relevant information first. For instance,

---

Box 2
Contraindications for performing EUS-FNA

Contraindication for endoscopic examination

    Cardiac or respiratory instability

    Suspected perforated viscus

    Nonfasting patient or undecompressed upper gastrointestinal obstruction

Coagulation disorder

    Anticoagulants

    Antiplatelet therapy[a]

Inaccessible lesion

    Lesion not visualized

    Large vessel or duct interposition

    Metastatic lesion with primary mass interposition

EUS-FNA results will not alter subsequent management

[a] Aspirin or nonsteroidal antiinflammatory drug use is not contraindicated.

in the setting of a pancreatic head mass with suspicious liver nodules, FNA of the liver lesions may provide a positive cytologic diagnosis and confirm that the patient is not a surgical candidate.

Position the Echoendoscope (as Straight as Possible)

Whenever possible, the echoendoscope should be straight. This makes needle movement easier and reduces the risks of damage to the accessory channel during insertion of the needle into the scope.

In our experience, most pancreatic lesions (including pancreatic head/uncinate lesion) can also be biopsied with the scope in a straight position. To do so, the scope should be passed into the second duodenum and then withdrawn into a "short" position. By withdrawing the scope toward the duodenal bulb, most pancreatic head lesions can be accessed and punctured. However, when withdrawn sufficiently, this position will become unstable, and the scope will slip into the stomach. Lesions near the pancreatic genu are often difficult to biopsy with this withdrawal technique because they often become visible just at the moment that the position becomes unstable.

For these lesions (and any other lesions that cannot be accessed with the scope in a straight position), it is necessary to assume a "long" position, with the scope in the bulb or prepyloric region. This position will also provide a mechanical advantage when trying to puncture indurated lesions in the pancreatic head region.

Select the Appropriate Needle

The 22g needle was used initially for EUS-FNA, but later 19g and then 25g needles became available. More recently, needles with a distal notch have gained favor for some authors.

There is growing consensus that the smaller needles, especially the 25g needle, are easier to use, produce less bloody samples, and increase the yield for malignancy.

Newer notched needles claim to more easily provide core samples and to improve the yield of cytologic specimens. Currently, the data are conflicting, and more randomized trials comparing these needles to standard needles are required.

For cytology, the authors use exclusively the 25g needle for all solid lesion EUS-FNA.

Insert the Needle into the Scope

If at all possible, the needle should be inserted into the scope with the scope in a straight position. Therefore, even if the lesion can only be accessed with the scope in a long position, it is best to withdraw the scope into a straight position, insert the needle, and then to reposition the scope for biopsy. One should never use excessive force to push the sheath past an excessive bend, as this could result in perforation of the inner lining of the biopsy channel. Instead, the echoendoscope should be withdrawn into a straight configuration before attempting to reinsert the needle system completely.

For lesions to be accessed from the second duodenum, the needle should be inserted into the scope only **after** the scope has been placed into the second duodenum. In other words, the duodenal sweep should not be negotiated with the needle and/or sheath protruding from the biopsy channel because there is a risk if duodenal laceration during this maneuver.

The rubber cap covering the operating channel must be removed before inserting the needle system. Once the needle is fully inserted into the echoendoscope, the base of the needle should be luer-locked to the operating channel (**Fig. 1**).

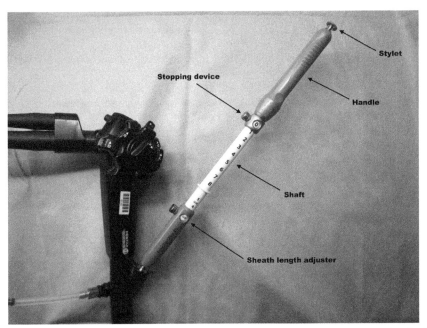

Fig. 1. The needle system is firmly luer-locked to the operating channel of the echoendoscope.

In some cases, the lesion to target may be less visible once the needle is in position; this can be explained either by artifact induced by the needle and/or sheath or by reducing the coupling between the gut wall and the ultrasound probe. Reducing the length of the sheath and applying suction to reduce air artifact between the ultrasound probe and the gut wall may help correct the problem. When using stiff, large caliber needles, increased rigidity of the scope may also alter its angulation, provoking less adequate images.

Position the Lesion in the Needle Path

Once the scope is in position, finer movements must be performed to bring the lesion into a position that will allow it to be punctured. Ideally, it should be positioned so that the lesion is within the natural path of the needle, so that minimal tip deflection and/or elevator deflection of the needle is needed (**Fig. 2**). If this is not possible, it should be

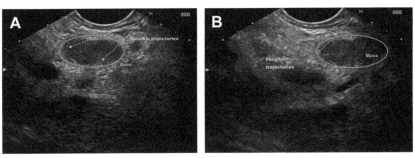

Fig. 2. (*A*, *B*) Correct positioning of a perigastric lymph node before FNA. (*A*) The lesion is within the natural path of the needle and elevator path. (*B*) Incorrect positioning.

positioned within the range of deflection provided by the elevator (**Fig. 3**). The elevator can be used to increase the angle between the needle and the ultrasound probe, but not to reduce it (**Fig. 4**).

Once this position is attained, it is best to lock the up-down control, so that the thumb can then be used to move the elevator, if needed.

Next, the needle sheath should be adjusted so that it protrudes just beyond the elevator. Most commercially available needles are manufactured with a sheath length adjuster. This device is located near the bottom of the needle shaft and allows the endosonographer to determine the proper length of sheath to exit the echoendoscope into the gut lumen (see **Fig. 1**). To minimize ultrasound artifacts caused by the shaft and to maximize elevator deflection capabilities, the needle sheath should be kept at a short distance from the operating channel exit. However, to avoid traumatizing the inner lining of the operating channel during needle deployment, one must be certain that the needle sheath terminates outside the operating channel (**Fig. 5**).

After needle sheath adjustment is performed, the screw must be tightly wound to avoid inadvertently advancing the sheath during needle thrusting, which could result in gut wall trauma. Needle sheath adjustment is usually performed when the needle is first used and rarely requires further manipulation during the subsequent passes.

A stopping device locks the needle inside the sheath, avoiding accidental injury or scope trauma during manipulation and insertion of the needle into the echoendoscope. Before puncturing the lesion, the stopping device must be unscrewed to allow needle deployment. The stopping device can be set so as to limit the maximum distance that the needle can travel (**Fig. 6**); this can be helpful in situations where inserting the needle beyond the limits of the target lesion would be dangerous (eg, the target lies directly over a vascular structure). Once the target lesion is in position on the screen, the caliper function can be used to measure the distance between the ultrasound probe and the desired area to sample. The stopping device can then be set to this distance.

To ensure maximum control, the fixed component of the needle handle should be grasped between the palm and the last 2 or 3 fingers of the right hand. The movable portion should be held between the thumb and index finger, which allows fine or vigorous needle movements to be performed, but with control. Any method that does not allow such control should be avoided (**Fig. 7**).

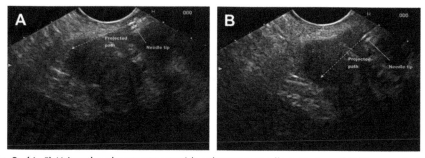

Fig. 3. (*A, B*) Using the elevator to provide adequate needle trajectory. (*A*) The needle is in its natural state with the elevator in neutral position, resulting in inadequate positioning. (*B*) Elevator use deflects the needle trajectory into a correct path.

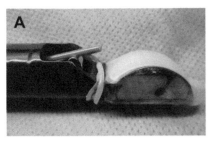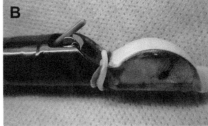

Fig. 4. (*A, B*) Elevator range of movement. (*A*) No elevator use. (*B*) Maximal deflection of elevator.

As discussed earlier, movement of the FNA needle is easier if it is straight. Any bend in the needle induced by excessively tipping up and/or torqueing the echoendoscope or by applying pressure with the elevator will increase resistance during needle deployment and may cause the needle to bend in an axis that will make it disappear from the ultrasound field of view. This situation is encountered most often when the EUS probe is placed in the duodenal bulb or the second duodenum.

To minimize risks of puncturing other vital structures, try to limit the distance the needle must travel to reach the target. One should avoid puncturing undrained, obstructed ducts that may provoke cholangitis or pancreatitis.

Should a structure such as a bile duct or blood vessel be punctured, it is logical to assume that the risk of leakage is lower if the needle enters perpendicular to the vessel/duct as opposed to passing tangentially and causing a linear laceration. Therefore, contact with all vessels should be avoided, but particularly when passing the

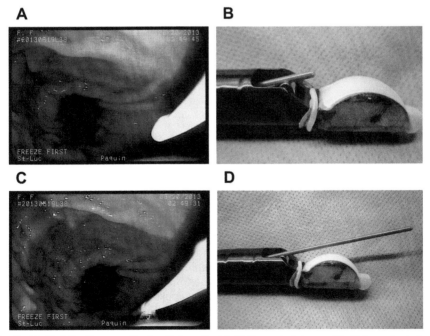

Fig. 5. (*A–D*) Adjusting needle sheath length. (*A, B*) Correct distance. (*C, D*) Excessively long distance.

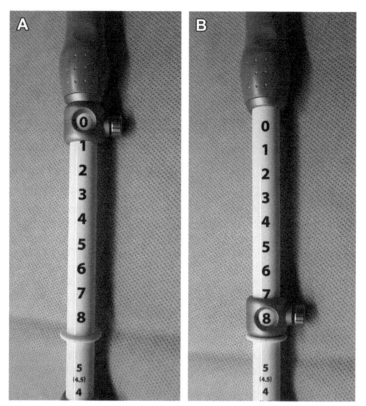

Fig. 6. (A, B) Stopper adjustment. (A) Stopper on. (B) Stopper off.

needle laterally to a vessel. Scanning the FNA path with power Doppler before needle insertion is a good way to exclude any unsuspected significant blood vessels in the targeted path.

Puncture the Lesion and Move the Needle Within the Lesion

Once the needle assembly and lesion are in adequate position, tissue sampling may begin. The needle should always be seen under real-time ultrasound guidance during tissue sampling to avoid traumatizing other structures. The goal is to insert the needle into the lesion, making repetitive back-and-forth thrusting movements into the lesion to shear off cells and collect them within the needle lumen; this requires that the needle be kept in the ultrasound-imaging plane and that thrusting movements be deliberate, always keeping an eye on the distal tip of the needle. Care should be taken to ensure that the needle does not exit the confines of the lesion during sampling. This will avoid contamination of the specimen with unwanted surrounding tissues.

Once the lesion is ready for puncture, sweeping the projected needle path with power Doppler to detect blood vessels can be performed. Before beginning to advance the needle, firm upward tip deflection should be applied using the up/down dial. This tends to bring the lesion closer to the echoendoscope and to reduce the tendency of the needle to push the ultrasound probe away from the gut wall, which can reduce the ultrasound image quality by allowing air to seep in between the probe and the gut wall. It also provides a mechanical advantage when trying to puncture an indurated lesion.

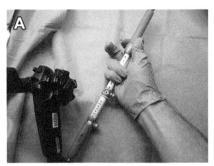
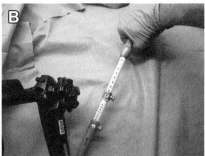
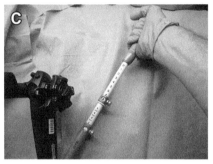

Fig. 7. (*A–C*) Holding the needle. (*A*) Correct positioning. (*B*) Incorrect method. (*C*) Another incorrect method.

Firm upward tip deflection also increases tension on the gut wall, thereby facilitating the puncture of mobile and thick walls such as the stomach body.

The needle should first be advanced approximately 1 cm out of the sheath, just enough to localize the tip in the ultrasound field. Once the tip has been identified, the elevator can be used to adjust the needle trajectory if needed. The needle can then be advanced into the lesion under ultrasound guidance.

If, for some reason, the needle tip can no longer be seen once the lesion has been punctured, all forward movement of the needle should be stopped. Continuing to advance the needle in the hope that the tip will become visible is a mistake and can result in inadvertent puncture of structures deep or lateral to the target lesion. Instead, the first reflex should be to slowly withdraw the needle; this will help localize the tip without risking puncture of deep structures. If this is ineffective, slow left and right movement of the shoulders can help bring the needle into the ultrasound imaging plane.

If both these techniques fail, the needle should be withdrawn completely from the lesion into the sheath. If it is possible that the scope position could have caused the needle to be bent, the needle assembly should be removed from the echoendoscope and the needle straightened if needed (see later discussion). The puncture can then be attempted again. This situation may be frequently encountered when the scope is torqued, especially in the duodenal bulb or sweep.

Once the needle is in the lesion and the tip clearly seen, the needle is moved back and forth several times within the lesion, with adequate force to produce cell shearing. Should needle thrusting reduce visibility by separating the transducer from the gut wall, slight forward pressure applied to the echoendoscope shaft will push the probe back against the wall. Constant gut lumen suctioning with the echoendoscope during needle deployment can also reduce any air seepage risk between the probe and gut wall.

Instead of sampling just one region of the lesion before processing the sample, the authors favor a "multi-pass" technique, which involves sampling widely through the lesion many times, before removing the needle from the scope. The needle is moved through the entire diameter of the lesion for 5 to 10 strokes, and the needle is withdrawn from the lesion and moved to a different region of the lesion. Approximately five regions per lesion are sampled before processing the sample. The multi-pass technique differs from the "fanning" technique in that the latter involves trying to sample different regions without removing the needle completely from the lesion (**Fig. 8**).

If the elevator deflection tip was used to adjust the needle angle, it may be helpful to return the elevator to the relaxed position once the needle is inside the lesion. This will allow the needle to move more freely.

Withdraw the Needle

After completing a pass, the needle should be completely withdrawn into the sheath. The locking device should be returned to its original upmost position and secured with the screw. To confirm complete needle withdrawal, the "0" numeral should be clearly seen within the locking device.

Process the Aspirate

This issue is addressed in further detail elsewhere in this issue. To avoid clotting in the needle, the aspirate should be expressed from the needle as quickly as possible. The authors expel all samples on to a glass slide using and air-filled syringe. The sample is then smeared using a second slide. This produces two slides per pass. If a cell block is required, a different sample is expelled with an air-filled syringe into a receptacle containing 10 cc of 50% alcohol.

If the needle is blocked, the aspirate can be forced out by inserting the stylet. Once the clot has been expressed on to a slide or container, the syringe should be used to express any remaining material from the needle.

Prepare the Needle for Subsequent Passes

The same needle can be used multiple times for several passes. A needle change may be required if it malfunctions or if the tip becomes too dull. If prior aspirates were bloody, rinsing the needle with normal saline before the next pass will wash out remaining debris.

If the needle is bent, it must be straightened before reinsertion into the scope. Otherwise, it will deflect out of the ultrasound plane during subsequent passes. To

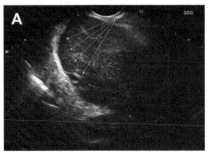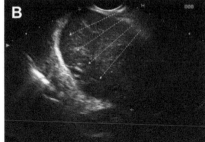

Fig. 8. (*A, B*) Sampling patterns. (*A*) Fanning technique. (*B*) Multipass technique.

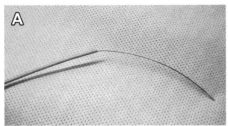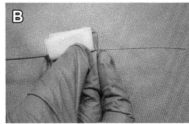

Fig. 9. (*A, B*) Straightening the needle. (*A*) Bent needle. (*B*) Straightening the needle.

straighten the needle, push it completely out of the sheath to expose it. Use your fingers to manually redress it (**Fig. 9**). An alcohol swab can then be used to clean the outer surface of the needle.

POTENTIAL MODIFICATIONS TO THE BASIC TECHNIQUE: STYLET, SUCTION

Traditionally, EUS-FNA was performed with the needle stylet in place during the initial puncture and with suction applied during needle movement.

There are multiple randomized trials showing that the stylet adds no benefit to EUS-FNA. Therefore, there is no available evidence justifying the use of the stylet, other than to help expel a specimen that may be clotted inside the needle.

There is also no convincing, reproducible evidence showing that any type of suction increases the yield for malignancy, but multiple studies have shown an undesirable increase in sample bloodiness.

Therefore, for cytology, the authors perform EUS-FNA with no stylet and no suction.

SUMMARY

1. For solid lesions, the basic EUS-FNA technique consists of proper positioning and moving of the needle inside the lesion with multiple to and fro movements under ultrasound guidance.
2. Many additions to the basic EUS-FNA technique have been described, but none appear to clearly improve the yield other than moving the needle effectively and in many different areas of the lesion.
3. For the goal of obtaining cytologic specimens, there is no clear advantage to use of the stylet, suction, larger diameter needles, or other modified needles.

REFERENCES

1. Dumonceau JM, Polkowski M, Larghi A, et al. Indications, results, and clinical impact of endoscopic ultrasound (EUS)-guided sampling in gastroenterology: European Society of Gastrointestinal Endoscopy (ESGE) Clinical Guideline. Endoscopy 2011;43:1–16.
2. ASGE Standards of Practice Committee, Anderson MA, Ben-Menachem T, et al. Management of antithrombotic agents for endoscopic procedures. Gastrointest Endosc 2009;70(6):1060–70.
3. Adler DG, Jacobson BC, Davila RE, et al. ASGE guideline: complications of EUS. Gastrointest Endosc 2005;61(1):8–12 [Erratum in Gastrointest Endosc 2005;61(3): 502].

Techniques for Endoscopic Ultrasound-Guided Fine-Needle Biopsy

Nikola Panic, MD[a,b], Alberto Larghi, MD, PhD[b],*

KEYWORDS

- Endoscopic ultrasonography • Fine-needle aspiration • Fine-needle biopsy
- Tissue acquisition • Histology • Core biopsy

KEY POINTS

- Although endoscopic ultrasound-guided fine-needle aspiration (EUS-FNA) is accurate, it cannot fully characterize certain neoplasms, and lack of cytology expertise may result in a limited perceived usefulness of EUS.
- EUS Tru-Cut biopsy does not offer any clear advantage compared with EUS-FNA and is technically demanding, with a low transduodenal yield.
- Standard 19-G and 22-G FNA needles with or without high negative pressure have proved to be reliable in obtaining high-quality histologic samples in various indications.
- The novel 19-G and 22-G ProCore needles (Cook Medical, Bloomington, IN, US) have shown a high yield in obtaining histologic samples, whereas 25-G ProCore seems unsuitable for histology.
- EUS-FNB is expected to refine differential diagnostic capabilities, favor widespread EUS use, and pave the road to targeted therapies and monitoring of treatment response.

INTRODUCTION

Since its initial description in 1992,[1] endoscopic ultrasound-guided fine-needle aspiration (EUS-FNA) has emerged as the procedure of choice to obtain samples to reach definitive diagnosis of lesions of the gastrointestinal (GI) tract and of adjacent organs.[2] Although EUS-FNA is accurate, especially when on-site cytopathology evaluation is available,[3–5] cytology does require a high degree of expertise rarely found outside high-volume tertiary-care centers.[6] This situation has created a barrier to the dissemination of EUS in the community and in many countries, because the lack of cytology expertise results in low diagnostic accuracy and therefore limits the overall usefulness of EUS.[7]

The obtainment of a tissue biopsy specimen for histologic examination may overcome this main limitation of EUS-FNA. A tissue core biopsy with preserved

[a] Digestive Endoscopy Unit, Catholic University, Largo A. Gemelli, 8, Rome 00168, Italy;
[b] Department of Medicine, University of Belgrade, Dr Subotica 8, Belgrade 11000, Serbia
* Corresponding author.
E-mail address: albertolarghi@yahoo.it

architecture is critical to diagnose and fully characterize certain neoplasms, such as lymphomas and GI stromal tumors. Moreover, tissue specimens for histologic examination also provide the opportunity (1) to easily immunostain the tissue, further increasing differential diagnostic capabilities; (2) to reach a specific diagnosis for benign diseases not always obtainable with a cytologic sample, thus sparing patients from more invasive and risky sampling procedures or costly and unnecessary follow-up examinations, and (3) to potentially perform tissue profiling or cell culture needed to guide targeted therapies for individualized treatment of patients with cancer of the GI tract.[8–10]

In the past, the ability to obtain fragments of tissue for histologic examination with FNA needles of various diameters had been tested,[11–13] and a Tru-Cut biopsy needle dedicated for EUS-guided fine-needle biopsy (EUS-FNB), the Quick-Core® needle (Cook Medical, Bloomington, IN, US), was developed but without meaningful advantages over EUS-FNA.[14–16] More recently, a new technique called EUS fine-needle tissue acquisition (EUS-FNTA), using standard 22-gauge and 19-gauge needles, has been developed and evaluated in few studies,[17–19] and a new needle, the ProCore needle (Cook Medical, Bloomington, IN, US), specifically designed to obtain histologic samples has become available and tested in clinical practice.[20–23] It is desirable that these new techniques and needles coupled with refinements in specimen processing will move the practice of EUS from cytology to histology, thereby facilitating the expansion of EUS use throughout the world.

This article reviews the EUS-FNB techniques developed so far, the clinical results, and their limitations as well as their future perspective.

EUS-GUIDED TRU-CUT BIOPSY
Background

Large-caliber cutting needles to acquire tissue core biopsy specimens with preserved architecture to allow for histologic examination have been used for many years to perform percutaneous (under conventional ultrasonographic or computed tomographic guidance), intraluminal (transanal, transrectal, transvaginal, transjugular), and surgical (laparoscopic, open) biopsies.[24–26] Based on these experiences, it appeared reasonable to translate this needle technology to develop a needle able to perform Tru-Cut biopsy under EUS guidance. In 2002, Wiersema and colleagues[27] presented the first experience using the Quick-Core, a 19-gauge needle capable of collecting an 18-mm tissue specimen sufficient for histologic examination. These investigators conducted a study in swine models reporting the safety and feasibility of EUS-guided Tru-Cut biopsy (EUS-TCB) using the Quick-Core needle that enabled histologic sampling from the liver, spleen, left kidney, and body of the pancreas through a transgastric approach.[27] A few months later, the same group reported the results of the first study in humans in which 19 patients with intestinal and extraintestinal lesions were evaluated.[28] Patients underwent both EUS-TCB and EUS-FNA. Overall, EUS-TCB was found to be more accurate than EUS-FNA (85% vs 60%), with a significantly reduced number of needle passes required for diagnosis (mean 2.0 vs 3.3, $P<.05$). No complications were encountered.

Since then, several studies have been conducted in order to examine the feasibility and safety of EUS-TCB, as well as to compare its performance with other EUS-guided sampling techniques.[14–16,29–46]

Design and Technique

The EUS-TCB device has a spring-loaded mechanism built into the handle of the needle, making possible automated acquisition of biopsy specimens (**Fig. 1**). The

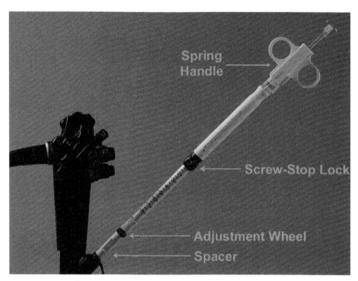

Fig. 1. Tru-Cut needle affixed to a linear echoendoscope demarcating the individual components of the handle portion of the device, including the following: spring-loaded mechanism built into the handle, which permits automated collection of a biopsy specimen; a screw-stop lock, which when unlocked allows advancement of the needle up to 8 cm and protects against inadvertent advancement; an adjustment wheel, which rotates the device into the proper orientation; and a spacer, which may be used, depending on the length of the linear echoendoscope by the manufacturer. (*Adapted from* Levy MJ, Wiersema MJ. EUS-guided trucut biopsy. Gastrointest Endosc 2005;62:418, with permission; and *Courtesy of* Mayo Clinic Foundation, Rochester, MN.)

handle also contains a screw-stop lock, which allows advancement up to 8 cm and an adjustment wheel, which rotates the device to orient into the proper position. The nonhandle portion consists of an outer catheter sheath, an internal 19-gauge cutting sheath, an 18-mm-long specimen tray, and a 5-mm-long stylet tip (**Fig. 2**). Before insertion in the working channel of the echoendoscope, the needle needs to be prepared in the firing position by retraction of the handle, which causes withdrawal of both the cutting sheath and the specimen tray. The needle is then advanced until the tip is nearly flush with the catheter sheath. After this preparation, the device is introduced in the working channel of the echoendoscope and screwed securely into the biopsy channel Luer-Lok adapter. In order to improve sampling collection, the device needs to be oriented by rotating the needle so that the 19-gauge marker on the handle is aligned with the model number on the echoendoscope. In this position, the specimen tray directly faces the transducer. Once the target lesion has been placed in the proper position, the needle is advanced under real-time EUS guidance, with all controls of the endoscope, including the elevator, released. The spring handle is then pressed forward, resulting in the advancement of the specimen tray into the target lesion, which is performed under continuous EUS monitoring. After at least 30 seconds, further pressure on the spring handle is applied, which fires the device and obtains a biopsy specimen. Once the procedure is completed, the screw-stop is locked and the needle removed from the echoendoscope.

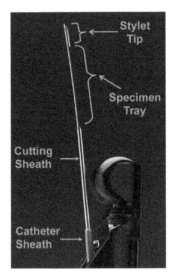

Fig. 2. Nonhandle portion of the Tru-Cut needle showing the following: outer catheter sheath; an internal 19-gauge cutting sheath, which shaves off the tissue specimen; an 18-mm-long specimen tray, which contains the tissue core; and a 5-mm-long stylet tip. (*Adapted from* Levy MJ, Wiersema MJ. EUS-guided trucut biopsy. Gastrointest Endosc 2005;62:418, with permission; and *Courtesy of* Mayo Clinic Foundation, Rochester, MN.)

Results

Table 1 summarizes the results of the published studies that have evaluated the performance of EUS-TCB in patients, with various indications. After the initial study by Levy and colleagues,[28] who evaluated a small group of patients with intestinal and extraintestinal lesions and reported that transgastric EUS-TCB was more accurate and required fewer passes than transgastric FNA, Larghi and colleagues[29] reported their experience in a cohort of patients with pancreatic solid masses. These investigators were able to collect pancreatic tissue samples in 74% of the patients, with a diagnostic accuracy of 87%. They showed a high rate of failures (40%) when the procedure was performed through the duodenum, thus reflecting the difficulty in using the device with the scope in a bent position. Similar failure rates for transduodenal puncture of pancreatic masses have been reported by Itoi and colleagues,[30] whereas Sakamoto and colleagues[32] reported a lower failure rate of 17%.

Subsequently, various studies have been published, most of which involved small patient populations and are not reviewed in detail (see **Table 1**). Three studies, including a meaningful number of patients, are available that evaluated the use of both EUS-TCB and EUS-FNA with different sampling strategy.[31,33,37] Wittmann and colleagues[31] evaluated 159 patients with a variety of solid lesions (83 pancreatic, 76 nonpancreatic) who underwent EUS-FNA alone (maximum 4 passes) in cases of lesions less than 2 cm in diameter and EUS-FNA followed by EUS-TCB (maximum 3 passes) for lesions with a diameter greater than 2 cm. A trend toward an increased number of adequate samples with the combination of both techniques versus EUS-FNA alone was found ($P = .056$), which was statistically significant if only nonpancreatic sites were considered ($P = .044$). No major complications for EUS-TCB were reported. The overall accuracy for FNA, TCB, and FNA plus TCB was 77%, 73%, and 91%, respectively. The combination of both sampling modalities versus EUS-FNA alone resulted in a significant improvement in accuracy ($P = .008$), which was mainly because of the additional value of EUS-TCB in sampling of nonpancreatic sites (EUS-FNA alone was 78%, EUS-TCB alone 83%, and EUS-FNA/TCB 95%, $P = .006$). These findings prompted the investigators to conclude that the combination of EUS-FNA/TCB can improve adequacy of sampling and diagnostic accuracy for lesions greater than 2 cm compared with either technique alone.[31]

Subsequently, Aithal and colleagues[33] compared the efficacy of a strategy of dual sampling (performing both FNA and TCB, 95 patients) with a strategy of sequential sampling (performing FNA only when TCB samples were macroscopically inadequate, 72 patients) in 167 patients with solid lesions. In 86% of the cases, the sampling procedure was performed through the esophagus or the stomach. The results of the dual sampling strategy revealed that the combined accuracy of EUS-FNA and EUS-TCB was significantly higher than that of FNA alone (92.6% vs 82.1%, $P = .048$), but not that of TCB alone (92.6% vs 89.5%, $P = .61$). Using the sequential sampling strategy, an accurate diagnosis was achieved in 92% of the patients, a rate similar to the 93% observed with the dual sampling strategy, suggesting that the former strategy could save the use of an additional needle, and thereby costs, in many patients.[33] One patient with mediastinal tuberculosis developed a cold abscess after EUS-TCB.

Berger and colleagues[37] in a retrospective study evaluated the performance of EUS-FNA followed by EUS-TCB in 70 consecutive patients with mediastinal lesions. The diagnostic accuracy of EUS-FNA, EUS-TCB, and both procedures combined did not differ significantly (93%, 90%, and 98%, respectively). No complications were observed. In 15 of the 20 patients with cytologic specimens showing malignancy, the diagnosis could be further specified with histologic analysis (tumor origin in 8, clear-cut lymphoma diagnosis in 4, and specification of tumor characteristics in 3). Despite these findings, the investigators suggested limiting the use of EUS-TCB to specific cases in which EUS-FNA was inconclusive.[37]

However, the study that assessed the performance of EUS-TCB in the largest patient population did not involve a comparison with EUS-FNA.[16] Of the 247 patients evaluated, 113 had pancreatic masses, 34 esophagogastric wall thickening, and 100 extrapancreatic lesions. A median of 3 needle passes per patient was performed, and in 14 of the 247 patients (6%), a technical failure occurred, which that in 57% of the cases was related to transduodenal puncture. The overall diagnostic accuracy was 75%, with a 2% complication rate. Independent predictors for a positive diagnostic yield were number of passes greater than 2 ($P = .05$) and the route of biopsy (stomach vs duodenum, $P = .001$; stomach vs esophagus, $P = .041$).[16]

Taking into consideration all the studies, no clear advantage for EUS-TCB over EUS-FNA has been shown (see **Table 1**), even in patients with suspected lymphomas or subepithelial lesions, which are considered a class IIa indication for the use of EUS-TCB.[47] In addition, the Tru-Cut needle is difficult to handle and the technique is less intuitive than EUS-FNA and is associated with an increased risk for complications. For these reasons, this technically demanding needle has failed to reach widespread use outside tertiary-care centers but is considered as the primer to future developments in EUS-FNB.

EUS-FNB USING A STANDARD 22-GAUGE NEEDLE
Background

In 2000, Voss and colleagues,[13] in an attempt to overcome some of the limitations of EUS-FNA, described their experience in obtaining tissue specimens from pancreatic masses using a standard 22-gauge FNA needle in association with high negative suction pressure by using a 30-mL syringe. These investigators were able to gather tissue

Table 1
Studies that evaluated the performance of the Quick-Core needle for EUS-TCB

Reference	No. of Patients	Patient Population	Yield EUS-TCB (%)	EUS-TCB Accuracy (%)	EUS-FNA Accuracy (%)	Yield of Transduodenal Biopsy (%)
Levy et al,[28] 2003	19	Intestinal and extraintestinal lesions	NA	85	60	NA
Larghi et al,[29] 2004	23	Pancreatic masses	74	61	NA	40
Varadarajulu et al,[14] 2004	18	Abdominal and mediastinal lesions	89	78	89	NR
Itoi et al,[30] 2005	16	Pancreatic masses	69	NR	NA	40
Wittmann et al,[31] 2006	96	Abdominal and mediastinal lesions	88	73	77	NR
Storch et al,[35] 2006	41	Abdominal and mediastinal lesions	NR	76	76	NA
Saftoiu et al,[34] 2007	30	Abdominal and mediastinal lesions	89	68	73	NA
Aithal et al,[33] 2007[a]	167	Abdominal and extra-abdominal masses	89	89	82	NR
Storch et al,[36] 2008	48	Lymph nodes, lung masses, esophageal wall masses	94	79	79	NA
Shah et al,[15] 2008	51	Pancreatic masses	86	52	89	NR
Sakamoto et al,[32] 2008[b]	24	Pancreatic masses	50	54	92	17
Berger et al,[37] 2009	70	Mediastinal lesions	94	90	93	NA
DeWitt et al,[39] 2009	21	Suspected hepatic parenchymal disease	100	90	NA	NA
Mizuno et al,[42] 2009	14	Suspected autoimmune pancreatitis	100	76	88	NR

Polkowski et al,[44] 2009	49	Gastric subepithelial lesions	63	89	NA	NA
Thomas et al,[16] 2009	247	Masses in pancreas, esophagogastric wall and extrapancreatic lesions	87	75	NA	NR[c]
Wahnschaffe et al,[45] 2009	24	Abdominal and extra-abdominal lesions	83	95	NA	NA
Ribeiro et al,[40] 2010	24	Suspected lymphomas	100	73[d]	0[d]	NA
DeWitt et al,[41] 2010	38	Suspected upper gastrointestinal or rectal gastrointestinal mesenchymal tumors	97	79	76	NA
Lee et al,[43] 2011	65	Gastric subepithelial lesions	57	NP	NP	NA
Mohamadnejad et al,[46] 2011	6	Extramural pelvic masses	83	80	NR	NA
Cho et al,[38] 2013	27	Mediastinal lesions	NR	67	78	NA

Abbreviations: NA, not applicable; NR, not reported.

[a] Patients with lesions that needed a transduodenal approach were included only when the lesion could be approached with the scope in a relatively straight position.

[b] FNA accuracy using 25-gauge needle.

[c] Site of biopsy (stomach vs duodenum vs esophagus) was identified as predictor of positive diagnostic yield.

[d] Accuracy for diagnosis and subclassification of lymphomas.

core specimens in 81% of the patients, with a diagnostic accuracy of 74.4%. Subsequently, other groups reported their experience in using a standard 22-gauge FNA needle with or without high negative suction pressure to obtain samples for histologic evaluation.[17,48–51] In particular, Larghi and colleagues[17] used the Alliance II system (Boston Scientific, Natick, MA) to obtain a high steady and continuous negative suction. They named their procedure EUS-FNTA to distinguish it from standard EUS-FNA.

Design and Technique

The EUS-FNTA technique with high negative pressure developed by Larghi and colleagues[17] is performed by using the Alliance II inflation system (**Fig. 3**), which is attached to a standard 22-gauge FNA needle. Once the needle is advanced in the target lesion under real-time EUS imaging, the stylet is withdrawn and the Alliance II system is attached to the proximal end of the needle. The Alliance II system is then turned into the suction mode, and a high negative continuous suctioning pressure corresponding to the 35-mL or 60-mL syringe, a value arbitrarily chosen, is applied. The lock of the syringe is then opened to apply steadily and continuously high negative suction pressure during the to-and-fro movements of the needle inside the target lesion.

Results

Results of studies evaluating the possibility of acquiring a tissue biopsy sample for histologic examination using a standard 22-gauge needle are summarized in **Table 2**.[13,17,48–51] Variable yield and diagnostic accuracy have been found in the different studies, the reason for which may be related to the different technique used and how the samples were handled. The group from Clichy, France[13] first reported the use of a standard 22-gauge needle to acquire tissue sample for histologic examination allowing analysis of tissue structure with serial section and the possibility to perform better immunostaining to increase diagnostic accuracy. To theoretically increase the possibility of acquiring a tissue sample, these investigators used high

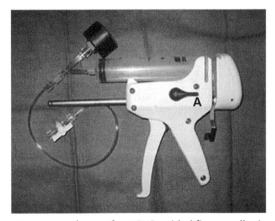

Fig. 3. The Alliance II system used to perform EUS-guided fine-needle tissue acquisition. This system was attached to the proximal end of a standard FNA needle and after turning it into the suction mode (A) was used to apply steady and high negative continuous suctioning at 35 mL of the 60-mL syringe. (*From* Larghi A, Noffsinger A, Dye CE, et al. EUS-guided fine needle tissue acquisition by using high negative pressure suction for the evaluation of solid masses: a pilot study. Gastrointest Endosc 2005;62:769; with permission.)

Table 2
Studies evaluating the possibility of acquiring a tissue biopsy sample for histologic examination using a standard 22-gauge needle

Reference	No. of Patients	Patient Population	Yield of Core Tissue (%)	Diagnostic Accuracy (%)
Voss et al,[13] 2000[a]	99	Pancreatic masses	81	68
Larghi et al,[17] 2005[b,c]	27	Solid masses	96	76.9
Iglesias-Garcia et al,[48] 2007	62	Pancreatic masses	83.9	88.7
Gerke et al,[51] 2009[b]	120	Solid masses and lymph nodes	27.8	77.8[d]
Moeller et al,[49] 2009	192	Pancreatic masses	86.5	71.4
Noda et al,[50] 2010	32	Solid masses and lymph nodes	NA	93.9

[a] Using high negative suction pressure with a 30-mL syringe.
[b] Using high negative suction pressure obtained using the Alliance II inflation system.
[c] Results obtained with a single needle pass for tissue acquisition was performed at the end of a standard FNA.
[d] Diagnostic accuracy calculated based on both histologic and cytologic specimens.

negative suction pressure by using a 30-mL syringe in a large cohort of patients with pancreatic solid lesions. Overall, the procedure was feasible in 90 of the 99 patients (90.9%), with the obtainment of material that could be analyzed for histology in 73 patients (81% of the patients in whom the procedure was feasible and 73.7% of the entire cohort, respectively), which was diagnostic in 67 patients (74.4% of the patients in whom the procedure was feasible and 67.7% of the entire cohort, respectively). Minor bleeding occurred in 5% of all cases, which was managed conservatively. Diagnostic accuracy was significantly better for adenocarcinomas than for neuroendocrine tumors (81% vs 47%, $P<.02$), although tumor size did not influence the results. This promising report was not followed by any other confirmatory or negative study until 5 years later, by Larghi and colleagues,[17] using a similar amount of negative suction pressure steadily applied through the use of the Alliance II inflation system in patients with solid masses. These patients included 27 with pancreatic, mediastinal, left adrenal, liver, gallbladder and gastric wall masses. All patients first underwent EUS-FNA, with a total of 5 passes performed. Using the same 22-gauge FNA needle, an extra pass was performed with the technique described earlier, and in all but 1 patient, a tissue specimen for histologic examination was procured, with no complications. EUS-FNA and EUS-FNTA reached the same diagnostic accuracy of 76.9% (in some patients with negative results at both procedures, a definitive diagnosis was not reached and the results were considered false negative), prompting the investigators to speculate that EUS-FNTA could perform better as the starting sampling technique.[17] However, this inference was partially disproved by the only other study that further investigated the role of this technique,[51] which involved mainly patients with enlarged lymph nodes, who represented 61% of the entire patient population studied. The content of the needle after EUS-FNTA was directly placed into formalin for histologic examination. Tissue core biopsy specimens were found in only 27.8% of the 36 patients evaluated. On the other hand, diagnostic accuracy was found to be 77.8%, a result similar to the one described by Larghi and colleagues,[17] thus implying that a sample for at least cytologic evaluation was obtained.

Without using high negative suction pressure, Iglesias-Garcia and colleagues[48] assessed the value of an extra pass performed using the same 22-gauge needle used for 2 previous FNA passes in obtaining tissue core specimens in 62 patients with pancreatic masses. Histologic samples were adequate in 83.9% of the cases, with a 6.5 ± 5.3 mm mean length of the retrieved core specimen. Overall, correct diagnosis from the samples collected at the third needle pass was 88.7%, meaning that a few samples had some cells that were sufficient to facilitate a cytologic diagnosis but not sufficient to render a histologic core for evaluation. In a subsequent study, Möller and colleagues[49] further investigated the capability of collecting tissue samples from 192 patients with pancreatic masses using a 22-gauge needle without high negative suction pressure. The material, which was retrieved by reinserting the stylet in the needle, was first visually evaluated for the presence of core specimens, which were subsequently carefully harvested by syringe suction and placed in formalin. The remaining liquid material was placed in saline solution or smeared onto glass slides for cytologic analysis. Using this technique, adequate samples for histologic evaluation were found in 85.9% of patients, with only 1 or 2 passes performed. An adequate cytologic specimen was also available in 93.2% of these cases. Overall, diagnostic accuracy was 71.4% and 77.6% for histologic and cytologic samples, respectively, with an extremely high accuracy of 87.5% when both histologic and cytologic results were combined.[49] Noda and colleagues[50] performed a similar study on 33 patients with pancreatic masses, in whom samples were half evaluated for cytology and half for histology by the cell-block method. Reading of the cell block was diagnostic in 25 of the 33 patients (75.8%) and in 31 of the 33 (93.9%) after immunostaining was performed.

EUS-FNB USING A STANDARD 19-GAUGE NEEDLE
Background

Between 2005 and 2006, 2 groups of Japanese investigators[30,52] first reported their experiences in using a standard 19-gauge needle to gather core biopsy specimens for histologic examination in patients with solid pancreatic masses and with mediastinal or intra-abdominal lymphadenopathy of unknown origin. These investigators reported an overall diagnostic accuracy of 68.8% and 98%, respectively. This discrepancy in the overall reported accuracy was caused by the high rate of failure (5 of 8 patients, 62.5%) of the sampling procedure when performed through the duodenum, as required for patients with pancreatic head and uncinate process masses.[30] However, the impressively high capability (88%) to correctly subtype lymphomas in patients with lymphadenopathy of unknown origin reported in the study by Yasuda and colleagues[52] clearly showed that tissue specimens acquired with a standard 19-gauge needle could have an important role in establishing a definitive diagnosis in selected patient populations.

Inspired by these promising results and in an attempt to overcome the limitation of the use of a standard 19-gauge needle through the duodenum, we modified the technique described by Itoi and colleagues[30] and by Yasuda and colleagues[52] by removing the stylet before insertion of the needle into the working channel of the EUS scope in order to increase needle flexibility and improve its performance.[18] This technique, which we continued to name EUS-FNTA to distinguish it from EUS-FNA, has been tested in different patient populations and in some specific cases, in which we believed a histologic sample could be more useful than a cytologic one to reach a definitive diagnosis.[18,19,53–55]

EUS-FNTA Technique

The EUS-FNTA technique is performed by using a disposable standard 19-gauge needle. The needle is prepared before insertion into the working channel of the echoendoscope by removing the stylet and attaching to its proximal end a 10-mL syringe already preloaded with 10 mL of negative pressure. The needle is then advanced under EUS guidance a few millimeters inside the target lesion. After opening the lock of the syringe to apply negative pressure, 2 or 3 to-and-fro motions inside the lesion using the fanning technique[56] are made, which together account for 1 needle pass. The needle is removed after closing the lock of the syringe and the collected specimens are placed directly in formalin by flushing the needle with saline and sent for histologic examination.

Results

Table 3 summarizes the results of all studies in which a standard 19-gauge needle has been used to gather samples for histologic analysis, independent of the technique used.[18,19,30,52–55,57–62] As shown in **Table 3**, apart from the study by Itoi and colleagues,[30] in which a high technical failure rate was found when the procedure was performed through the duodenum, the overall technical success and yield in all the published studies were higher than 90%. Moreover, overall diagnostic accuracy was also found to be higher than 90%, with the only exception of the study by Iwashita and colleagues,[57] in which patients with a pancreatic mass suspicious for autoimmune pancreatitis (AIP) were evaluated. In the latter study, although specimens for histologic analysis were obtained in 93% of the patients, a definitive histologic diagnosis of AIP based on lymphoplasmacytic infiltration around pancreatic ducts, obliterative phlebitis, or positive IgG4 immunostaining was possible in only 43% of the cases. In the remaining 50% of the patients with available tissue for histologic analysis, specific histologic findings of AIP could not be found, and a diagnosis of idiopathic chronic pancreatitis was made.[57] This low diagnostic yield can be attributed to the patchy distribution of the specific histologic changes of AIP,[63] thus rendering the amount of tissue obtained with EUS-guided biopsy insufficient to establish a definitive diagnosis. On the other hand, in all patients with available tissue, a malignant cause could be excluded, which is important in order to safely start empirical therapy for AIP with steroids.[57]

After the first publication in 2006,[52] the Japanese group from Gifu University Hospital published their subsequent experiences in patients with mediastinal lymphadenopathy and a clinical presentation suggestive of sarcoidosis[58] and in a larger cohort of patients with mediastinal or abdominal lesions suspicious for lymphoma.[59] Both studies showed the value of using a standard 19-gauge needle to (1) confirm the clinical suspicion of sarcoidosis[58] and (2) to establish a diagnosis of lymphoma with subclassification in a high percentage of patients, thus sparing them from more invasive diagnostic procedures.[59] These results suggest that a 19-gauge needle should be used as the sampling procedure of choice in these patient populations.

In our first experience using the modified EUS-FNTA technique, besides patients with lymphadenopathy of unknown origin, we also evaluated patients with subepithelial lesions, esophagogastric wall thickening, and with pancreatic body or tail solid lesions after a negative FNA, in whom we deemed histologic samples to be more appropriate than cytologic aspirates.[18] Overall, in the cohort of 120 patients consecutively enrolled, the procedure was technically successful in all but 1 patient without any complications, with a diagnostic yield of 96.7% and a diagnostic accuracy of 93.2%. Specimens gathered with the EUS-FNTA helped make not only a diagnosis of malignancy but also a definitive diagnosis of a benign disease in 20 patients who were spared from more invasive diagnostic procedures and from unnecessary follow-up examinations.[18] Representative cases of benign and malignant diagnoses are shown in **Fig. 4**. In this first experience, we decided not to enroll patients with pancreatic head/uncinate masses after a negative FNA, because of the fear that the

Table 3
Studies evaluating the possibility of acquiring a tissue biopsy sample for histologic examination using a standard 19-gauge needle

Reference	No. of Patients	Patient Population	Technical Success (%)	Yield (%)	Diagnostic Accuracy (%)
Itoi et al,[30] 2005[a]	16	Pancreatic masses	81	68.8	68.8
Yasuda et al,[52] 2006	104	Mediastinal or abdominal lymphadenopathy	100	100	98.1; 88 accuracy in subclassification of lymphoma
Iwashita et al,[58] 2008	41	Mediastinal lymphadenopathy suspicious for sarcoidosis	100	95.1	95.1
Larghi et al,[18] 2011[b,c]	120	Heterogeneous patient population	99.2	96.7	93.2
Larghi et al,[19] 2012[c]	30	Pancreatic masses suspicious for nonfunctional neuroendocrine neoplasia	100	93.3	93.3
Iwashita et al,[57] 2012	44	Pancreatic masses suggestive of autoimmune pancreatitis	100	93	43.2
Yasuda et al,[59] 2012	152	Mediastinal or abdominal lesions suspicious for lymphoma	97	97	93.4; 95 accuracy in subclassification of lymphoma (142 patients)
Varadarajulu et al,[62] 2012	38	Pancreatic masses/ subepithelial lesions	100	94.7	94.7
Stavropoulos et al,[60] 2012[d]	31	Patients with abnormal liver tests undergoing EUS to rule out biliary obstruction	100	91	91
Eckardt et al,[61] 2012	46	Gastric subepithelial lesions	—	59	52
Larghi et al,[53] 2013 (unpublished data)[e,c]	121	GI subepithelial lesions	99.2	93.4	93.4

[a] All failures occurred when sampling was performed from the duodenum.
[b] Consecutive patients with subepithelial lesions, esophagogastric wall thickening, mediastinal and abdominal masses/lymphadenopathy of unknown origin, pancreatic body or tail lesions after a negative FNA were included in the study.
[c] The EUS-FNTA technique was used.
[d] Adequate specimen defined as a length of 15 mm with the presence of at least 6 portal tracts.
[e] All procedures were performed using the forward viewing EUS scope.

presence of a stent, which is usually placed after EUS-FNA, could interfere with the procedure.[18] Subsequently, we performed a second study in patients with pancreatic lesions suspicious for nonfunctional neuroendocrine neoplasia (NF-NEN).[19] In these patients, we performed Ki-67 proliferation index determination, which can be better

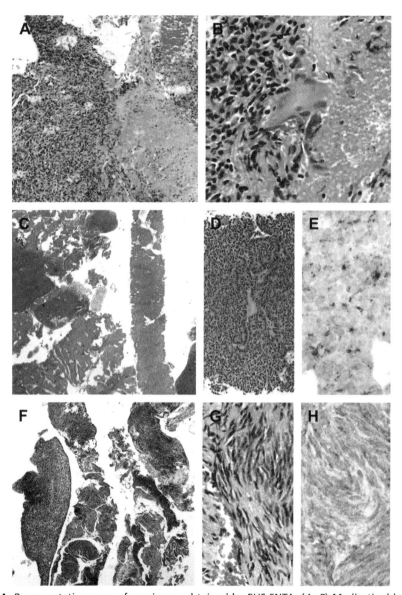

Fig. 4. Representative cases of specimens obtained by EUS-FNTA. (*A, B*) Mediastinal lymph node: (*A*) abundant tissue fragments, at higher magnification (*B*) showing caseous material (*left part of the micrograph*) and polynucleated giant cells consistent with a tubercular granuloma, as also later confirmed by polymerase chain reaction methods; hematoxylin-eosin. (*C–E*) Body-tail of the pancreas: (*C, D*) multiple large tissue fragments of a well-differentiated, nonfunctioning, neuroendocrine tumor, with a typical trabecular structure, low-grade histology void of necrosis and mitotic figures (*D*) and chromogranin A expression at immunohistochemistry (*E*); (*C, D*) hematoxylin-eosin; (*E*) immunoperoxidase. (*F–H*) Peri-gastric lesion: (*F*), abundant, large fragments of neoplastic tissue with solid structure, in absence of necrosis, composed of regular, fused cell with mild atypia (*G*) intensely immuno-reactive for c-Kit and consistent gastrointestinal stromal tumor; (*F, G*) hematoxylin-eosin; (*H*) immunoperoxidase. (*From* Larghi A, Verna EC, Ricci R, et al. EUS-guided fine-needle tissue acquisition by using a 19-gauge needle in a selected patient population: a prospective study. Gastrointest Endosc 2011;74:507; with permission.)

determined on tissue biopsy specimens and has an important prognostic value on management decisions.[19] Thirty consecutive patients with a pancreatic mass with a mean diameter of 16.9 ± 6.1 mm were enrolled. The lesions were located throughout the pancreas, including the pancreatic head and uncinate process (8 patients, representing 27% of the cohort), which could be approached only from the duodenum. The procedure was technically successful in all cases, and in 28 of the 30 patients, a specimen for histologic examination was retrieved and confirmed the suspicious diagnosis of NF-NEN. Moreover, in 26 patients (92.9% of those with an available specimen and 86.6% of the entire cohort), Ki-67 determination could be performed (**Fig. 5**). Comparison with the Ki-67 determination on surgical specimens, which represents the gold standard, was feasible in 12 patients and showed an agreement in 10 cases when a cutoff of more than 2% to define G2 tumors was applied. Conversely when a cutoff of 5% was used, which is suggested to be more useful than the 2% value to stratify prognosis of patients with pancreatic NF-NEN,[64,65] an agreement was found in all patients.[19] These results indicate that preoperative Ki-67 determination on EUS-FNTA specimens may be used for the discussion with a patient regarding the available therapeutic options.

Two other patient populations in whom the use of a standard 19-gauge needle has been evaluated are patients with abnormal liver tests of unclear cause referred for EUS to exclude biliary obstruction and those with subepithelial lesions.[53,60,61] In the first patient population, after an unrevealing EUS, Stavropoulos and colleagues[60] investigated the value of EUS-guided liver biopsy performed in the same session using a standard 19-guage needle. An adequate specimen was defined as a specimen that was at least 15 mm long and with at least 6 complete portal tracts. Among the 22 patients evaluated, a specimen with these characteristics could be retrieved in 20 (91%), which was diagnostic in all cases. There were no procedural complications, including 5 higher-risk patients with relative coagulopathy (platelets <100,000/μL, international normalized ratio >1.3). In patients with subepithelial lesions, 2 studies have reached opposite conclusions reporting a diagnostic accuracy of 52%[61] versus 93.4%.[53] The reason for this discrepancy is unclear. We speculated that in our study,[53] the use of the EUS-FNTA technique with removal of the stylet before the procedure, which renders the needle more flexible and easy to operate, coupled with the utilization of the forward viewing therapeutic linear echoendoscope, which seems to ensure easier deployment of a 19-gauge needle,[66–68] could account for the better results reported. With the specimens we collected (representative cases are shown in **Fig. 6**), we were able to perform genetic analysis for diagnostic purposes in 3 patients in whom immunohistochemical studies were negative, despite histopathologic features that were suggestive of gastrointestinal stromal tumor (GIST). The capability of performing genotype profiling of GISTs is relevant beyond its diagnostic significance, because it has a prognostic impact and allows optimizing chemotherapy for unresectable cases and for other selected cases in which neoadjuvant therapy may be a useful option.[69,70]

Varadarajulu and colleagues[62] recently published their experience of using a newly developed flexible 19-gauge needle (Expect 19 Flex, Boston Scientific, Natick, MA) made of nitinol, which is supposed to have a better performance for transduodenal puncture. These investigators evaluated 32 patients with pancreatic head/uncinate masses or peripancreatic masses approached from the duodenum and 6 patients with subepithelial lesions in the stomach (5) and in the rectum (1). On-site cytopathology evaluation and cell-block analysis were performed. The procedure was successful in all patients, and examination of cell-block specimens showed optimal histologic core tissue in 36 of 38 (93.7%) patients, which was

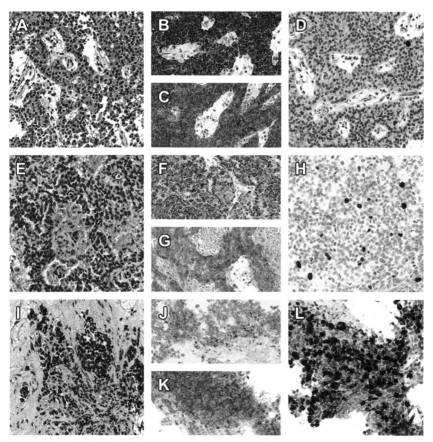

Fig. 5. Examples of grading for neuroendocrine neoplasms in EUS-FNTA samples. (*A–D*) Grade 1 primitive neuroectodermal tumor (p-NET) showing trabecular histology, mild atypia (*A*), intense immunoreactivity for chromogranin A (*B*) and synaptophysin (*C*) and rare cells with nuclear labeling for Ki-67 (*D*). (*E–H*) Grade 2 p-NET showing large trabecular structure, moderate cell atypia (*E*), intense immunoreactivity for chromogranin A (*F*) and synaptophysin (*G*) and discrete cells with nuclear labeling for Ki-67 (*H*). (*I–L*) High-grade, grade 3, pancreatic neuroendocrine carcinoma fragmented sample showing abundant desmoplasia and solid islets of cells with severe atypia and scarce cytoplasm (*I*), focal and often faint immunoreactivity for chromogranin A (*J*), intense and diffuse immunoreactivity for synaptophysin (*K*), and diffuse nuclear labeling for Ki-67 (*L*). (*A, E, I*) hematoxylin-eosin; (*B–D, F–H* and *J–L*) immunoperoxidase. (*From* Larghi A, Capurso G, Carnuccio A, et al. Ki-67 grading of nonfunctioning pancreatic neuroendocrine tumors on histologic samples obtained by EUS-guided fine-needle tissue acquisition: a prospective study. Gastrointest Endosc 2012;76:575; with permission.)

diagnostic in all cases. Based on these results[62] and a report by Itoi and colleagues,[71] the same group proposed an algorithm in which, in centers where an on-site cytopathologist is not available, they recommended to perform EUS-FNB instead of EUS-FNA by using a standard 19-gauge needle for lesions approached from the esophagus, stomach, and rectum, and to use the flex 19-gauge needle for transduodenal puncture.[72] In our opinion, there are insufficient data to make this suggestion, and further experiences with this needle are necessary before a definitive conclusion on the value of the proposed algorithm can be drawn.

EUS-FNB USING PROCORE NEEDLES

Introduction

Although the Quick-Core needle failed to reach widespread use because of technical difficulty associated with its use and the relative lack of advantages over standard FNA needles, the same manufacturer developed a new needle with a different design, the ProCore needle.[20] To meet all the needs and have a needle to cover for different clinical scenarios and level of difficulty, 3 needle sizes have been developed: the 19-gauge, the 22-gauge, and the 25-gauge ProCore needles.

Design and Technique

All ProCore needles are 1.705 m long, made of stainless steel with a nitinol stylet. The stylet that runs through the cannula of the needle matches the bevel tip. There is a lateral opening of varying length depending on the needle size (**Fig. 7**; **Table 4**), which presents a reverse bevel to hook and cut the tissue, entrapping it into the needle. This

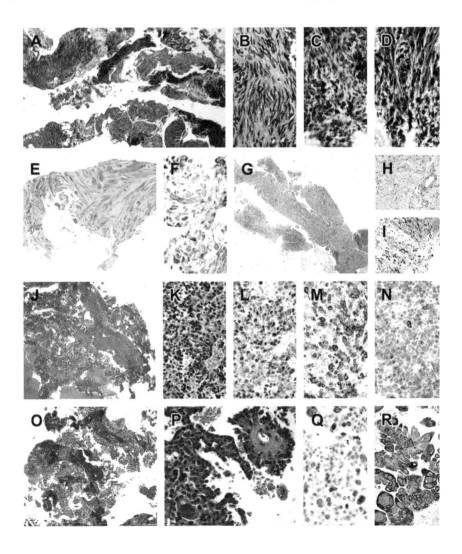

Table 4 Main characteristics of the different available ProCore needles			
	ECHO-HD-25-C	ECHO-HD-22-C	ECHO-HD-19-C
Needle outer diameter (mm)	0.56	0.71	1.07
Needle inner diameter (mm)	0.37	0.51	0.94
Needle length (m)	1.705	1.705	1.705
Needle bevel	Lancet	Lancet	Lancet
Stylet tip design	Lancet	Recessed ball	Recessed ball
Reverse bevel length (mm)	2	2	4
Distance of the needle tip from the reverse bevel (mm)	3	3.9	5
Sheath size (Fr)	5.2	5.2	4.8
Needle material	Stainless steel	Stainless steel	Stainless steel
Stylet material	Nitinol	Nitinol	Nitinol

reverse bevel is located at a different distance from the tip of the needle, depending on the needle size (see **Fig. 7**; **Table 4**). Characteristics and differences between ProCore needles are shown in **Table 4**.

In the first published study,[20] which involved 5 European centers, each participating center used a different sampling technique. At univariate and multivariate analyses, the only variable associated with the obtainment of an optimal sample for histologic analysis and to make a correct final diagnosis was the intervention of an experienced

Fig. 6. Representative cases of tissue type and amount obtained by EUS-FNTA in subepithelial lesions. (*A–D*) Gastrointestinal stromal tumor (GIST): abundant tissue fragments (*A*) at higher magnification showing a spindle cell neoplasm (*B*) with a strong and diffuse immune positivity for CD117 (*C*) and DOG1 (*D*), which unequivocally qualified as a GIST (*A, B,* hematoxylin-eosin; *C,* CD117 IHC; *D,* DOG1 IHC; original magnification: *A* ×20, *B, C,* and *D* ×400). (*E, F*) Esophageal leiomyoma. The abundance of the available fragments allowed not only to detect the presence of spindle cells with abundant eosinophilic cytoplasm with bland nuclei and no mitotic activity but also to appreciate their arrangement in intersecting fascicles (*E*); these findings, together with an intense desmin reactivity (*F*) in the absence of staining with CD117 and DOG1 (not shown) led to a straightforward diagnosis of leiomyoma (*E,* hematoxylin-eosin; *F,* desmin IHC; original magnification: *E* ×200, *F* ×400). (*G–I*) Gastric schwannoma: the bioptic specimen showed a spindle cell neoplasm (*G, H*); the preservation of architectural details such as the presence of hyaline thickening of vessel walls (*H*) and the diffuse S-100 positivity (*I*) in the absence of CD117 and DOG1 staining (*not shown*) were diagnostic for a schwannoma (*G, H,* hematoxylin-eosin; *I,* S-100 IHC; original magnification: *G* ×40, *H, I* ×400). (*J–N*) Gastric metastasis of melanoma: the bioptic sample was composed of fragments of highly cellular neoplasm composed of atypical epithelioid cells (*J, K*) intensely and diffusely positive for S-100 (*L*), HMB-45 (*M*) and Melan-A (*N*), typical features of melanoma (*J, K,* hematoxylin-eosin; *L,* S-100 IHC; *M,* HMB-45 IHC; *N,* Melan-A IHC; original magnification: *J,* ×40, *K, L, M, N* ×400). (*O–R*) Gastric metastasis of ovarian serous papillary carcinoma: the bioptic fragments showed a neoplasm composed of epithelioid cells with marked atypia arranged in papillae (*O, P*), with nuclear WT1 immunoreactivity (*Q*) and intense staining for cytokeratin 7 (*R*) (*O, P,* hematoxylin-eosin; *Q,* WT1 IHC; *R,* cytokeratin 7 IHC; original magnification: *O* ×20, *P, Q, R* ×400). (*Data from* Larghi A, Fuccio L, Chiarello G, et al. EUS-guided fine-needle tissue acquisition in a large cohort of patients with subepithelial lesions using the forward viewing linear echoendoscope. Endoscopy, in press.)

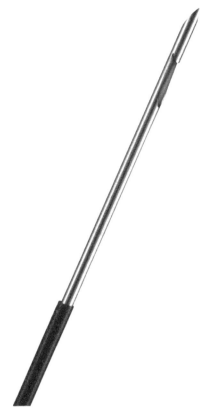

Fig. 7. Detailed image of the tip of the ProCore™ 19-gauge needle showing the notch with the reverse bevel technology for acquisition of tissue samples for histologic examination. (*From* Iglesias-Garcia J, Poley JW, Larghi A, et al. Feasibility and yield of a new EUS histology needle: results from a multicenter, pooled, cohort study. Gastrointest Endosc 2011;73:1189–96.)

pathologist to evaluate the sample. Site of the puncture (duodenum vs other sites), use or not of the stylet, number of to-and-fro movements (3–4 vs 1), number of needle passes (2–3 vs 1), and modality of sample retrieval (air, stylet, or saline solution) did not have any impact on tissue sample acquisition.[20] In a subsequent study from the same European group,[21] a standardized sample acquisition protocol was developed and performed as follows: (1) the needle was advanced into the target lesion under EUS guidance; (2) once inside the lesion, the stylet was removed and negative suction pressure was applied using a 10-mL syringe for 30 seconds; (3) 3 to-and-fro movements within the lesion were made; (4) suction was then released by closing the lock of the syringe and the needle was removed. Tissue samples were recovered in formalin or CytoLyt by flushing the needle with saline.[21]

A different sampling technique, the slow pull technique, has been proposed for the tissue acquisition procedure performed using the 25-gauge ProCore needle.[23] With this technique, once the needle is inside the lesion, the negative suction pressure is obtained by slowly and continuously pulling out the stylet from the needle while 10 to 20 to-and-fro movements are performed. Preliminary results[73] have reported this technique to result in a significantly higher yield compared with the suction method used in both the European ProCore studies.[20,21]

Results

The performance of the 19-gauge ProCore needle in the diagnosis of intraintestinal and extraintestinal lesions was evaluated in a multicenter study by Iglesias-Garcia and colleagues.[20] Among 109 patients with 114 heterogeneous lesions, EUS-FNB using this newly developed biopsy needle was technically feasible in 112 cases (98.24%), with no complications. The only 2 technical failures occurred when the sampling procedure was performed through the duodenum, accounting for an overall success rate of 94.3% (33/35) for transduodenal sampling. In both patients, who respectively had an aortocava lymph node and a pancreatic head tumor, failure was a result of the impossibility of removal of the stylet from the needle once inside the lesion. Overall, in all lesions in which the procedure was technically successful, a sample suitable for pathologic evaluation was obtained, which was adequate for histologic examination in 102 lesions (89.5%) and for cytologic evaluation in the remaining 10 cases (sample was processed as a cell block). Diagnostic accuracy was 86% for all lesions and 92.9% for malignant lesions, respectively. The only factor that positively correlated with a significant increase in the potential for establishing a definitive histologic diagnosis was the involvement of an expert pathologist.[20]

A study evaluating the interobserver agreement in grading the quality of specimens obtained with the 19-gauge ProCore needle among 5 expert pathologists from the 5 participating centers was performed.[74] Overall, an excellent interobserver agreement in the assessment of the histologic material was found among the involved pathologists, and this was particularly high (91.2%) with regard to sample adequacy, with a Fleiss κ that was 0.73 (95% confidence interval 0.61–0.81).[74] Moreover, when the same samples were evaluated by nonexpert pathologists, the interobserver agreement substantially decreased (unpublished data), thus suggesting the paramount importance of a pathologist dedicated to read EUS samples. It is our opinion that efforts to establish pathology expertise by combining their educational activities with those of endosonographers should be strongly encouraged.

The same study group subsequently evaluated the performance of the 22-gauge ProCore needle in a cohort of 61 patients with pancreatic masses, which in 57.4% of the cases were localized in the pancreatic head/uncinate, thus requiring a transduodenal approach.[21] Only 1 needle pass was performed using the protocol described earlier. In 1 patient with an uncinate process mass, the procedure failed because of inability to extend the needle out of the working channel of the echoendoscope. In the remaining patients with a successful sampling procedure, tissue specimens for histologic examination were retrieved in 55 (90.2%), which in all but 1 patient (88.5%) were judged adequate to make a definitive diagnosis. All adequate specimens were found to be diagnostic, thus accounting for an overall accuracy of 88.5%. These promising results prompted another group to design a randomized trial to compare the capability of this needle with that of a standard 22-gauge FNA needle in the obtainment of cytologic and histologic samples in 56 patients with pancreatic masses.[22] No significant difference in the median number of passes required for establishing on-site diagnosis, rates of diagnostic accuracy, or technical failure between the FNA and FNB needles was detected. Moreover, no significant difference between the 2 groups was found in the proportion of samples in which histologic core tissue was present (FNA 100% vs FNB 83.3%, $P = .26$).[22] On the other hand, histologic core of optimal quality was present in 66.7% of FNA specimens and 80% of FNB specimens ($P = .66$).[22] In a study with a similar design that included not only pancreatic masses but also other type of lesions such as lymph nodes and intraintestinal and extraintestinal lesions, the 22-gauge ProCore required significantly fewer needle passes compared with a standard 22-gauge FNA needle to achieve adequacy.[75] Despite similar cytologic interpretability, diagnostic accuracy, and amount of cell-block material between the 2 needles, this finding can result in less procedural time and cost savings.[75] Future multicenter studies in large patient populations with heterogeneous indications are needed to better clarify if the 22-gauge ProCore has any advantage over a standard 22-gauge FNA needle.

Iwashita and colleagues[23] reported the first experience in using the 25-gauge ProCore needle for the evaluation of 50 consecutive patients with solid pancreatic lesions. These investigators applied the slow pull technique described earlier. After FNB, the obtained material was expressed onto a glass slide by reinsertion of the stylet and any visible core was lifted off and placed in formalin, and smears for on-site cytopathologic evaluation were made from the residual material. The investigators found an impressively high sensitivity (83%) for cytologic diagnosis on the first pass, which increased to 91% and 96% at the second and third pass, respectively. On the first pass, in which the histologic analysis was performed on a per-pass basis, a sensitivity of 63% was found. This value increased to 87% at the subsequent 2 to 4 passes. The presence of a histologic core was found in only 12% of the patients after the first needle pass and in 32% of the patients at the subsequent 2 to 4 passes. In our opinion, these results indicate that the 25-gauge ProCore needle is a proficient needle to gather diagnostic cytologic specimen, probably even more efficient than a standard 25-gauge FNA needle, but cannot be used when a tissue core biopsy specimen is required to make the diagnosis.

SUMMARY AND FUTURE PERSPECTIVE

In the last decade, in an attempt to overcome some of the limitations of EUS-FNA, alternative sampling techniques and dedicated needles to obtain core tissue biopsy specimens for histologic examination under EUS guidance have been developed and tested, with varying success. These efforts may lead to a shift in this field from cytology to histology, which is easier to interpret, thus potentially contributing to the widespread utilization of EUS in the community and in countries where it may be difficult to develop cytology expertise. Moreover, in the era of individualized medicine, this shift will likely pave the road to targeted therapies and better approaches to the treatment of most GI malignancies, because tissue samples for histologic examination are more suitable for performing predictive molecular markers or cell culture with chemosensitivity testing to guide individualized therapies. This situation will transform diagnostic EUS into a more therapeutic procedure that not only gives a diagnostic answer but also offers the possibility to deliver the best treatment of individual patients. Based on these premises, we need to change our way of thinking and search for the right technique or the right needle that will give enough tissue to perform all studies to reach the diagnosis and to allow for personalized treatment of individual patients. This needle should be able to meet not only the needs of experts but also those of all individual endosonographers. We firmly believe that a close collaboration between endosonographers and pathologists is of paramount importance to succeed in this balanced effort to develop the right EUS-FNB needle/technique and should be strongly encouraged.

REFERENCES

1. Vilmann P, Jacobsen GK, Henriksen FW, et al. Endoscopic ultrasonography with guided fine needle aspiration biopsy in pancreatic disease. Gastrointest Endosc 1992;38:172–3.

2. Dumonceau JM, Polkowski M, Larghi A, et al. European Society of Gastrointestinal Endoscopy. Indications, results, and clinical impact of endoscopic ultrasound (EUS)-guided sampling in gastroenterology: European Society of Gastrointestinal Endoscopy (ESGE) Clinical Guideline. Endoscopy 2011;43:897–912.

3. Hébert-Magee S, Bae S, Varadarajulu S, et al. The presence of a cytopathologist increases the diagnostic accuracy of endoscopic ultrasound-guided fine needle aspiration cytology for pancreatic adenocarcinoma: a meta-analysis. Cytopathology 2013;24:159–71.

4. Iglesias-Garcia J, Dominguez-Munoz JE, Abdulkader I, et al. Influence of on-site cytopathology evaluation on the diagnostic accuracy of endoscopic ultrasound-guided fine needle aspiration (EUS-FNA) of solid pancreatic masses. Am J Gastroenterol 2011;106:1705–10.

5. Eloubeidi MA, Tamhane A, Jhala N, et al. Agreement between rapid onsite and final cytologic interpretations of EUS-guided FNA specimens: implications for the endosonographer and patient management. Am J Gastroenterol 2006; 101:2841–7.

6. Jhala NC, Jhala DN, Chhieng DC, et al. Endoscopic ultrasound-guided fine-needle aspiration. A cytopathologist's perspective. Am J Clin Pathol 2003;120: 351–67.

7. Kalaitzakis E, Panos M, Sadik R, et al. Clinicians' attitudes towards endoscopic ultrasound: a survey of four European countries. Scand J Gastroenterol 2009;44: 100–7.

8. Braat H, Bruno M, Kuipers EJ, et al. Pancreatic cancer: promise for personalised medicine? Cancer Lett 2012;318:1–8.

9. Wakatsuki T, Irisawa A, Terashima M, et al. ATP assay-guided chemosensitivity testing for gemcitabine with biopsy specimens obtained from unresectable pancreatic cancer using endoscopic ultrasonography-guided fine-needle aspiration. Int J Clin Oncol 2011;16:387–94.

10. Brais RJ, Davies SE, O'Donovan M, et al. Direct histological processing of EUS biopsies enables rapid molecular biomarker analysis for interventional pancreatic cancer trials. Pancreatology 2012;12:8–15.

11. Harada N, Kouzu T, Arima M, et al. Endoscopic ultrasound-guided histologic needle biopsy: preliminary results using a newly developed endoscopic ultrasound transducer. Gastrointest Endosc 1996;44:327–30.

12. Binmoeller KF, Thul R, Rathod V, et al. Endoscopic ultrasound-guided, 18-gauge, fine needle aspiration biopsy of the pancreas using a 2.8 mm channel convex array echoendoscope. Gastrointest Endosc 1998;47:121–7.

13. Voss M, Hammel P, Molas G, et al. Value of endoscopic ultrasound guided fine needle aspiration biopsy in the diagnosis of solid pancreatic masses. Gut 2000; 46:244–9.

14. Varadarajulu S, Fraig M, Schmulewitz N, et al. Comparison of EUS guided 19-gauge Trucut needle biopsy with EUS-guided fine-needle aspiration. Endoscopy 2004;36:397–401.

15. Shah SM, Ribeiro A, Levi J, et al. EUS-guided fine needle aspiration with and without trucut biopsy of pancreatic masses. JOP 2008;9:422–30.

16. Thomas T, Kaye PV, Ragunath K, et al. Efficacy, safety, and predictive factors for a positive yield of EUS-guided Trucut biopsy: a large tertiary referral center experience. Am J Gastroenterol 2009;104:584–91.

17. Larghi A, Noffsinger A, Dye CE, et al. EUS-guided fine needle tissue acquisition by using high negative pressure suction for the evaluation of solid masses: a pilot study. Gastrointest Endosc 2005;62:768–74.

18. Larghi A, Verna EC, Ricci R, et al. EUS-guided fine-needle tissue acquisition by using a 19-gauge needle in a selected patient population: a prospective study. Gastrointest Endosc 2011;74:504–10.

19. Larghi A, Capurso G, Carnuccio A, et al. Ki-67 grading of nonfunctioning pancreatic neuroendocrine tumors on histologic samples obtained by EUS-guided fine-needle tissue acquisition: a prospective study. Gastrointest Endosc 2012;76:570–7.

20. Iglesias-Garcia J, Poley JW, Larghi A, et al. Feasibility and yield of a new EUS histology needle: results from a multicenter, pooled, cohort study. Gastrointest Endosc 2011;73:1189–96.

21. Larghi A, Iglesias-Garcia J, Poley JW, et al. Feasibility and yield of a novel 22-gauge histology EUS needle in patients with pancreatic masses: a multi-center prospective cohort study. Surg Endosc 2013;27:3733–8.

22. Bang JY, Hebert-Magee S, Trevino J, et al. Randomized trial comparing the 22-gauge aspiration and 22-gauge biopsy needles for EUS-guided sampling of solid pancreatic mass lesions. Gastrointest Endosc 2012;76:321–7.

23. Iwashita T, Nakai Y, Samarasena JB, et al. High single-pass diagnostic yield of a new 25-gauge core biopsy needle for EUS-guided FNA biopsy in solid pancreatic lesions. Gastrointest Endosc 2013;7:909–15.

24. Hatada T, Ishii H, Ichii S, et al. Diagnostic value of ultrasound-guided fine-needle aspiration biopsy, core-needle biopsy, and evaluation of combined use in the diagnosis of breast lesions. J Am Coll Surg 2000;190:299–303.

25. Rodriguez LV, Terris MK. Risks and complications of transrectal ultrasound guided prostate needle biopsy: a prospective study and review of the literature. J Urol 1998;160:2115–20.

26. DurupScheel-Hincke J, Mortensen MB, Pless T, et al. Laparoscopic four-way ultrasound probe with histologic biopsy facility using a flexible tru-cut needle. Surg Endosc 2000;14:867–9.

27. Wiersema MJ, Levy MJ, Harewood GC, et al. Initial experience with EUS-guided trucut needle biopsies of perigastric organs. Gastrointest Endosc 2002;56:275–8.

28. Levy MJ, Jondal ML, Clain J, et al. Preliminary experience with an EUS guided trucut biopsy needle compared with EUS-guided FNA. Gastrointest Endosc 2003;57:101–6.

29. Larghi A, Verna EC, Stavropoulos SN, et al. EUS-guided trucut needle biopsies in patients with solid pancreatic masses: a prospective study. Gastrointest Endosc 2004;59:185–90.

30. Itoi T, Itokawa F, Sofuni A, et al. Puncture of solid pancreatic tumors guided by endoscopic ultrasonography: a pilot study series comparing Trucut and 19-gauge and 22-gauge aspiration needles. Endoscopy 2005;37:362–6.

31. Wittmann J, Kocjan G, Sgouros SN, et al. Endoscopic ultrasound-guided tissue sampling by combined fine needle aspiration and trucut needle biopsy: a prospective study. Cytopathology 2006;17:27–33.

32. Sakamoto H, Kitano M, Komaki T, et al. Prospective comparative study of the EUS guided 25-gauge FNA needle with the 19-gauge Trucut needle and 22-gauge FNA needle in patients with solid pancreatic masses. J Gastroenterol Hepatol 2009;24:384–90.

33. Aithal GP, Anagnostopoulos GK, Tam W, et al. EUS-guided tissue sampling: comparison of "dual sampling" (Trucut biopsy plus FNA) with "sequential sampling" (Trucut biopsy and then FNA). Endoscopy 2007;39:725–30.

34. Saftoiu A, Vilmann P, Guldhammer SB, et al. Endoscopic ultrasound (EUS)-guided Trucut biopsy adds significant information to EUS-guided fine-needle

aspiration in selected patients: a prospective study. Scand J Gastroenterol 2007;42:117–25.

35. Storch I, Jorda M, Thurer R, et al. Advantage of EUS Trucut biopsy combined with fine-needle aspiration without immediate on-site cytopathologic examination. Gastrointest Endosc 2006;64:505–11.

36. Storch I, Shah M, Thurer R, et al. Endoscopic ultrasound-guided fine-needle aspiration and trucut biopsy in thoracic lesions: when tissue is the issue. Surg Endosc 2008;22:86–90.

37. Berger LP, Scheffer RC, Weusten BL, et al. The additional value of EUS-guided Tru-cut biopsy to EUS guided FNA in patients with mediastinal lesions. Gastrointest Endosc 2009;69:1045–51.

38. Cho CM, Al-Haddad M, Leblanc JK, et al. Rescue endoscopic ultrasound (EUS)-guided Trucut biopsy following suboptimal EUS-guided fine needle aspiration for mediastinal lesions. Gut Liver 2013;7:150–6.

39. Dewitt J, McGreevy K, Cummings O, et al. Initial experience with EUS-guided Tru-cut biopsy of benign liver disease. Gastrointest Endosc 2009;69:535–42.

40. Ribeiro A, Pereira D, Escalón MP, et al. EUS-guided biopsy for the diagnosis and classification of lymphoma. Gastrointest Endosc 2010;71:851–5.

41. DeWitt J, Emerson RE, Sherman S, et al. Endoscopic ultrasound-guided Trucut biopsy of gastrointestinal mesenchymal tumor. Surg Endosc 2011;25:2192–202.

42. Mizuno N, Bhatia V, Hosoda W, et al. Histological diagnosis of autoimmune pancreatitis using EUS-guided trucut biopsy: a comparison study with EUS-FNA. J Gastroenterol 2009;44:742–50.

43. Lee JH, Choi KD, Kim MY, et al. Clinical impact of EUS-guided Trucut biopsy results on decision making for patients with gastric subepithelial tumors ≥ 2 cm in diameter. Gastrointest Endosc 2011;74:1010–8.

44. Polkowski M, Gerke W, Jarosz D, et al. Diagnostic yield and safety of endoscopic ultrasound-guided trucut biopsy in patients with gastric submucosal tumors: a prospective study. Endoscopy 2009;41:329–34.

45. Wahnschaffe U, Ullrich R, Mayerle J, et al. EUS-guided Trucut needle biopsies as first-line diagnostic method for patients with intestinal or extraintestinal mass lesions. Surg Endosc 2009;23:2351–5.

46. Mohamadnejad M, Al-Haddad MA, Sherman S, et al. Utility of EUS-guided biopsy of extramural pelvic masses. Gastrointest Endosc 2012;75:146–51.

47. Levy MJ, Wiersema MJ. EUS-guided Trucut biopsy. Gastrointest Endosc 2005; 62:417–26.

48. Iglesias-Garcia J, Dominguez-Munoz E, Lozano-Leon A, et al. Impact of endoscopic ultrasound-guided fine needle biopsy for diagnosis of pancreatic masses. World J Gastroenterol 2007;13:289–93.

49. Möller K, Papanikolaou IS, Toermer T, et al. EUS-guided FNA of solid pancreatic masses: high yield of 2 passes with combined histologic-cytologic analysis. Gastrointest Endosc 2009;70:60–9.

50. Noda Y, Fujita N, Kobayashi G, et al. Diagnostic efficacy of the cellblock method in comparison with smear cytology of tissue samples obtained by endoscopic ultrasound-guided fine-needle aspiration. J Gastroenterol 2010;45:868–75.

51. Gerke H, Rizk MK, Vanderheyden AD, et al. Randomized study comparing endoscopic ultrasound-guided Trucut biopsy and fine needle aspiration with high suction. Cytopathology 2010;21:44–51.

52. Yasuda I, Tsurumi H, Omar S, et al. Endoscopic ultrasound-guided fine needle aspiration biopsy for lymphadenopathy of unknown origin. Endoscopy 2006;38: 919–24.

53. Larghi A, Fuccio L, Chiarello G, et al. EUS-guided fine needle tissue acquisition in a large cohort of patients with subepithelial lesions using the forward viewing linear echoendoscope. Endoscopy, in press.

54. Larghi A, Lococo F, Ricci R, et al. Pleural tuberculosis diagnosed by EUS-guided fine-needle tissue acquisition. Gastrointest Endosc 2010;72:1307–9.

55. Larghi A, Lugli F, Sharma V, et al. Pancreatic metastases from a bronchopulmonary carcinoid diagnosed by endoscopic ultrasonography-guided fine-needle tissue acquisition. Pancreas 2012;41:502–4.

56. Bang JY, Magee SH, Ramesh J, et al. Randomized trial comparing fanning with standard technique for endoscopic ultrasound-guided fine-needle aspiration of solid pancreatic mass lesions. Endoscopy 2013;45:445–50.

57. Iwashita T, Yasuda I, Doi S, et al. Use of samples from endoscopic ultrasound-guided 19-gauge fine-needle aspiration in diagnosis of autoimmune pancreatitis. Clin Gastroenterol Hepatol 2012;10:316–22.

58. Iwashita T, Yasuda I, Doi S, et al. The yield of endoscopic ultrasound-guided fine needle aspiration for histological diagnosis in patients suspected of stage I sarcoidosis. Endoscopy 2008;40:400–5.

59. Yasuda I, Goto N, Tsurumi H, et al. Endoscopic ultrasound-guided fine needle aspiration biopsy for diagnosis of lymphoproliferative disorders: feasibility of immunohistological, flow cytometric, and cytogenetic assessments. Am J Gastroenterol 2012;107:397–404.

60. Stavropoulos SN, Im GY, Jlayer Z, et al. High yield of same-session EUS-guided liver biopsy by 19-gauge FNA needle in patients undergoing EUS to exclude biliary obstruction. Gastrointest Endosc 2012;75:310–8.

61. Eckardt AJ, Adler A, Gomes EM, et al. Endosonographic large-bore biopsy of gastric subepithelial tumors: a prospective multicenter study. Eur J Gastroenterol Hepatol 2012;24:1135–44.

62. Varadarajulu S, Bang JY, Hebert-Magee S. Assessment of the technical performance of the flexible 19-gauge EUS-FNA needle. Gastrointest Endosc 2012;76:336–43.

63. Zamboni G, Lüttges J, Capelli P, et al. Histopathological features of diagnostic and clinical relevance in autoimmune pancreatitis: a study on 53 resection specimens and 9 biopsy specimens. Virchows Arch 2004;445:552–63.

64. Scarpa A, Mantovani W, Capelli P, et al. Pancreatic endocrine tumors: improved TNM staging and histopathological grading permit a clinically efficient prognostic stratification of patients. Mod Pathol 2010;23:824–33.

65. Rindi G, Falconi M, Klersy C, et al. TNM staging of neoplasms of the endocrine pancreas: results from a large international cohort study. J Natl Cancer Inst 2012;104:764–77.

66. Larghi A, Lecca PG, Ardito F, et al. Evaluation of hilar biliary strictures by using a newly developed forward-viewing therapeutic echoendoscope: preliminary results of an ongoing experience. Gastrointest Endosc 2009;69:356–60.

67. Trevino JM, Varadarajulu S. Initial experience with the prototype forward-viewing echoendoscope for therapeutic interventions other than pancreatic pseudocyst drainage (with videos). Gastrointest Endosc 2009;69:361–5.

68. Larghi A, Seerden TC, Galasso D, et al. EUS-guided therapeutic interventions for uncommon benign pancreaticobiliary disorders by using a newly developed forward-viewing echoendoscope (with videos). Gastrointest Endosc 2010;72:213–5.

69. Corless CL, Barnett CM, Heinrich MC. Gastrointestinal stromal tumours: origin and molecular oncology. Nat Rev Cancer 2011;11:865–78.

70. Eisenberg BL, Smith KD. Adjuvant and neoadjuvant therapy for primary GIST. Cancer Chemother Pharmacol 2011;67(Suppl 1):S3–8.
71. Itoi T, Tsuchiya T, Itokawa F, et al. Histological diagnosis by EUS-guided fine-needle aspiration biopsy in pancreatic solid masses without on-site cytopathologist: a single-center experience. Dig Endosc 2011;23(Suppl 1):34–8.
72. Bang JY, Ramesh J, Trevino J, et al. Objective assessment of an algorithmic approach to EUS-guided FNA and interventions. Gastrointest Endosc 2013; 77(5):739–44.
73. Iwashita T, Nakai Y, Samarasena JB, et al. Endoscopic ultrasound-guided fine needle aspiration and biopsy (EUS-FNAB) using a novel 25-gauge core biopsy needle: optimizing the yield of both cytology and histology. Gastrointest Endosc 2012;75:AB183.
74. Petrone MC, Poley JW, Bonzini M, et al. Interobserver agreement among pathologists regarding core tissue specimens obtained with a new endoscopic ultrasound histology needle: a prospective multicentre study in 50 cases. Histopathology 2013;62:602–8.
75. Witt BL, Adler DG, Hilden K, et al. A comparative needle study: EUS-FNA procedures using the HD ProCore(™) and EchoTip(®) 22-gauge needle types. Diagn Cytopathol 2013. http://dx.doi.org/10.1002/dc.22971.

Tips to Overcome Technical Challenges in EUS-guided Tissue Acquisition

Peter Vilmann, MD, DSc[a], Andrada Seicean, MD, PhD[b],*,
Adrian Săftoiu, MD, PhD, MSc[a,c]

KEYWORDS

- Endoscopic ultrasound (EUS) • Fine needle aspiration (FNA) • Tissue acquisition
- EUS-FNA technique • EUS guided biopsy

KEY POINTS

- Tissue acquisition is necessary to guide the management of digestive diseases.
- Several tips and tricks are useful to overcome technical challenges in EUS-guided FNA procedures.

BACKGROUND

Endoscopic ultrasound-guided fine needle aspiration (EUS-FNA) is routinely performed to diagnose and stage pancreaticobiliary, esophageal, gastric, and rectal malignancies, as well as evaluate gastrointestinal subepithelial lesions and mediastinal and intra-abdominal lymphadenopathy. The reported accuracy rates of EUS-FNA vary and range from 71% to 98% for pancreatic masses, 85% to 90% for lymph nodes, and 67% to 92% for gastrointestinal subepithelial lesions.[1]

Nevertheless, the diagnostic yield of EUS-FNA depends on several factors, such as the experience of the endosonographer, the characteristics of the lesion, the clinical

Funding Sources: This work was supported by the research grant "Minimal invasive assessment of angiogenesis in pancreatic cancer based on imaging methods and molecular techniques (Angio-Pac)" Ideas programme, 164/2011, NRC-UEFISCDI, project number PN-II-ID-PCE-2011-3-0589, Romania.
Conflict of Interests: P. Vilmann has disclosures related to consultancy at Medi-Globe GmbH, Grassau, Germany (EUS needles); A. Seicean, Nil; A. Săftoiu, Nil.

[a] Department of Endoscopy, Gastrointestinal Unit, Copenhagen University Hospital, Herlev Ringvej 75, Herlev 2730, Denmark; [b] Department of Gastroenterology, Regional Institute of Gastroenterology and Hepatology, University of Medicine and Pharmacy, Croitorilor Street 19-21, Cluj-Napoca 400162, Romania; [c] Department of Gastroenterology, Research Center of Gastroenterology and Hepatology, Craiova, Romania
* Corresponding author.
E-mail address: andradaseicean@yahoo.com

status of the patient, the size and type of needle being used, the methods of specimen processing, and expertise of the cytopathologist.[2] Several tips and tricks are necessary to overcome the technical challenges of EUS-FNA.

PROBLEMS RELATED TO THE LESION AND ITS SURROUNDINGS
Difficult Location of Lesions

Whenever an EUS-guided biopsy is attempted, the position of the transducer in relation to the lesion is of major importance. The endoscope should always be advanced to a position that brings the transducer as close to the lesion as possible. However, there are some technical challenges related to the lesion and its surroundings that may influence the biopsy procedure. The most difficult regions to be reached by the echoendoscope are the deep part of the uncinate process, the second duodenum, the gastric fornix, and near the greater curvature. Other lesions, such as adjacent ulcers, scars, or diverticula, impede the best visualization of the lesion, and consequently subsequent EUS-guided puncture. One special situation is when the papilla is situated inside a diverticula. By using water instillation, it is frequently possible to visualize the papillary and suprapapillary regions. Avoiding puncture of vessels and pancreatic ducts should always be attempted (**Fig. 1**). Lesions located in the hepatoduodenal ligament or its surroundings in particular may pose a challenge because of an interposed vessel, such as the portal vein or the hepatic artery or its branches (**Fig. 2**). Fortunately, it is often possible to find an adequate window to perform an FNA without the presence of intervening vasculature or ductal structures. Before the procedure, anticoagulants should be stopped for 5 days and antiaggregants (eg, clopidogrel) should be stopped for for 5 to 7 days.[2]

Characteristics of Lesions

The characteristics of a lesion that is targeted during FNA influences the diagnostic results to a high degree. Diagnostic success is affected in particular if a lesion is hard and fibrotic, such as in solid pancreatic masses. The same is the case in lesions that are highly mobile, such as small submucosal tumors in the stomach. The best location for tumor sampling is thought to be the periphery of the tumor. The central part of the pancreatic tumor should be avoided because of extensive necrosis. The presence of acute pancreatitis, necrosis, or severe chronic pancreatitis with coexisting fibrosis could be misinterpreted as perfusion defects during contrast enhancement[3] or may be mistaken for cancer during elastography.[4] Although these

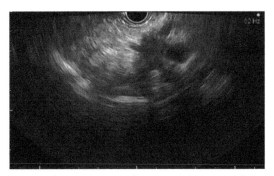

Fig. 1. Hypoechoic mass in the pancreatic isthmus with invasion of the splenic vein, portal confluence, and superior mesenteric vein. The FNA needle should avoid puncturing the vessels and the main pancreatic duct.

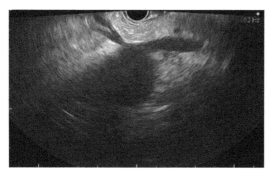

Fig. 2. Tumor in the pancreatic head invading the splenomesenteric confluence, which makes FNA technically difficult using the current position of the echoendoscope.

techniques could guide the tissue sampling, their incremental value has not been established yet. The presence of chronic pancreatitis features was associated with a lower accuracy of EUS-FNA for the differential diagnosis of pancreatic masses (73% vs 91%) and might need a higher number of passes for establishing the diagnosis.[5] The presence or absence of stents (either plastic or metallic) usually does not impede EUS-FNA,[6-8] although some suggest better outcomes when the stent is placed just 1 day before performing EUS-FNA.[7]

Most other authors have shown that there is no difference in diagnostic accuracy when a lesion is more than or less than 3 cm in diameter.[9] However, a single study has shown that the size of the tumor may be a restrictive factor in reaching an adequate diagnosis, especially for tumors less than 1 cm, where the sensitivity was found to be as low as 40%.[10] Concerning the tumors of 1 to 2, 2 to 3, 3 to 4, and greater than 4 cm, the diagnostic sensitivity was 75.9, 86.9, 93.2, and 91.6%, respectively.[10] The presence of intratumoral anechoic foci may require a higher number of passes.[11]

Aspiration from the edge of the lymph node (compared with the center) did not increase the likelihood of a correct diagnosis.[12] Coagulation necrosis within a lymph node on EUS was described as an ill-defined, rounded, and nonshadowing echogenic area. It is different from the linear, nonshadowing, hilar echogenic structure that may be seen in the center of benign lymph nodes and has a 70% accuracy for diagnosing malignancy on FNA.[13]

The results of a retrospective study on 107 patients showed that targeting the cyst wall of cystic lesions of the pancreas produces an increasing diagnostic accuracy of up to 56%.[14]

Impaired Passage or Altered Anatomy

The presence of an esophageal stricture can preclude echoendoscope passage. Then, either dilation or the use of miniprobe/slim scopes may be proposed. Miniprobes or nonoptic radial endoscopes enable only diagnostic evaluation, thus to perform FNA, a slim, linear echoendoscope or an endobronchial echoendoscope could be the answer. The endobronchial ultrasound videoscope with a thinner diameter than the conventional echoendoscope (6.2 mm instead of 12.8 mm) has been used successfully in several cases to guide FNA.[15-17] The main limitation is the impossibility to reach the head of the pancreas because the working length of this endoscope is too short. The lack of insufflation can be resolved by manual air insufflation that enables advancement of the scope and decreases the risk of esophageal perforation.[16]

The presence of food or fluid inside the esophagus or stomach, due to either an esophageal or a pyloric or duodenal stenosis, may impede the examination. In this case, the procedure should be postponed and the patient kept on a liquid diet for 2 to 3 days.

Previous surgery, a dominant pancreatic mass, or a duodenal stenosis may prevent the echoendoscope from reaching the second part of the duodenum. In most situations, the FNA can be performed from the duodenal bulb, with the help of an assistant, to maintain the scope position, or from the antrum, with much care to avoid vessels when targeting pancreatic head lesions. The main limitations are the view of the head of the pancreas after Roux-en-Y surgery. Nevertheless, in one study, most patients were able to get a complete pancreaticobiliary examination, including FNA, after Billroth II and Whipple surgeries, provided that the afferent limb could be intubated.[18] Deflecting the tip of the echoendoscope at the level of anastomosis increases the visual field for sonographic examination.

PROBLEMS RELATED TO ENDOSCOPE AND NEEDLE
Inadequate EUS Imaging

A successful biopsy specimen is dependent foremost on adequate EUS imaging so that the position of the needle can be monitored at all times. There are several factors that may impair optimal ultrasonic visualization, such as problems with balloon inflation, air in front of the transducer either due to air in the balloon or in the lumen, impaired acoustic coupling, or endoscope torquing.

It is rarely necessary to fill the balloon with water before or during EUS-guided biopsy. However, in a few indications this may be needed, either to anchor the transducer in the duodenum or to optimize needle visualization during biopsy. The presence of air in the balloon represents a technical problem that may impair the examination. In this situation, aspiration of the balloon content and subsequent refilling may solve the problem but often complete removal of the echoendoscope is necessary to remove the air bubbles completely from within the balloon. The presence of the needle inside the working channel may impede supplementary air suction, especially for nontherapeutic linear echoendoscopes with a thin working channel. If there is an accumulation of air in front of the targeted lesion, the procedure cannot be continued, because of the lack of visual control of the needle at the puncture site.

There are several situations in which the endoscopist has to torque or bend the echoendoscope, thus making the FNA difficult or impossible. The first situation is encountered in the second portion of the duodenum, where the tip of the endoscope is angulated and the needle exit for targeting lesions in the head of the pancreas or distal common bile duct is sometimes challenging. If the needle is forced to exit, the transducer might be damaged by accidental puncture. This damage could be avoided by having the sheath of the needle in the endoscopic view or by seeing the needle tip in the ultrasound view. For transduodenal targeting of the lesions, shortening of the echoendoscope is the best course of action. FNA can be performed safely with the help of an assistant to maintain the position of the echoendoscope. However, if a periduodenal compressive lesion limits straightening of the echoendoscope, then the position of the scope is maintained, the deflection of the tip of the scope is loosened, and the needle is advanced until it is in endoscopic view. The tip of the echoendoscope is then deflected again so as to bring the lesion within the trajectory of the needle. Air suction also helps to bring the gut wall closer to the probe.

The second situation in which torquing of the echoendoscope may impede FNA is the location of a lesion in the gastric fundus. If attempts to reach the lesion from the level of cardia fail, the needle must be advanced out of the working channel with the echoendoscope in a straight position before the scope is looped to reach the lesion.

A third situation in which torquing of the echoendoscope may influence FNA is in the stomach, due to the large gastric volume and the mobile gastric wall. When a lesion inside the gastric wall is targeted and biopsy is difficult or unsuccessful, one possibility is to attempt a 2-step puncture: the first step is to puncture the wall; the second step is then to target the lesion itself. Another possibility is to advance the scope further into the stomach to form a long loop, against the opposite gastric wall, so that the tip of the scope acts as a hinge.[19] Rapid (sharp) movements of the needle during transgastric FNA is preferable to avoid "bouncing" of the needle due to gastric mobility.

Choice of Needle

Currently, there are several types of needles for FNA and biopsy (histologic analysis): 22 G, 19 G, and 25 G. The choice of needle is based on various considerations such as the potential for complications, adequacy of specimen, and cost.[20–41]

The most commonly used needle is a 22 G, which is flexible and enables cytologic assessment without a significant risk for complications, although a 2% risk of acute pancreatitis was reported in a large retrospective series.[20] Nevertheless, hard lesions are sometimes better penetrated with the 25-G needle, which is thinner and easier to use in the distal duodenum (uncinate process) or to access lesions farther away from the transducer.[19,21] For uncinate process lesions, the use of the 22-G needle has been reported to be unsuccessful in up to 33% of cases.[22] Experimental laboratory simulations that compare resistance to needle advancement have shown that only the 22-G and 25-G needles are suitable for insertion into the target regions if tight angulation is present.[23]

The diagnostic accuracy for pancreatic masses when using the 22-G needles is up to 95%[24] and as low as 68% for subepithelial lesions.[25] A meta-analysis that compared the 22-G and 25-G needles for FNA of pancreatic and peripancreatic masses showed nonsignificant differences in sensitivity (78% vs 91%), specificity (100%), and complications (**Table 1**). Repeating the EUS-FNA in the case of initial negative cytology increases the yield of diagnosis.[28–30]

The overall rates of diagnostic adequacy for sampling pancreatic masses for cytology using the 22-G needle are variable compared with histology (82%–93% vs 84%–87%).[23] The overall diagnostic accuracy for histology on each pass is only 60% for the 25-G needle and 75% for the 22-G neeedle.[23] Histology showed a trend for superiority over cytology only in characterizing nonadenocarcinoma tumor types or inflammatory masses with a diagnosis being established in 90% to 100% of cases.[31–33] For submucosal lesions, the adequacy of FNA for histology is reported to be 43% to 100%.[34–36] The European Society of Gastrointestinal Endoscopy (ESGE) recommends routine procurement of tissue for histology when sampling subepithelial lesions.[2]

The 19-G aspiration needles are more rigid and transduodenal biopsies are difficult and sometimes impossible to use[41–44]; thus, their use is not routinely recommended.[2] The diagnostic accuracy for body/tail pancreatic lesions was shown to be superior when using 19-G needles compared with 22-G needles, offering more cytologic material in some circumstances.[42,43] A large step forward when using the 19-G needle is the ability to procure histology samples that offer more information about the diagnosis of rare tumors, metastases, lymphomas, and tumor differentiation for neuroendocrine tumors or subepithelial lesions.[45] However, there seems to be no advantage for the 19-G needles over 22-G needles for sampling subepithelial lesions.[46,47] In a large multicenter European study, it was feasible to use the 19-G FNA needle in

Table 1
Adequacy of cytologic diagnosis for comparative use of different size needles

Author, Year	No of Patients	Type of Study	Needle Used	Accuracy of Diagnosis for Cytology
Yusuf et al,[20] 2009	302 (pancreatic mass)	Retrospective	25 G	84% (Sensitivity)
	540 (pancreatic mass)		22 G	92% (Sensitivity)
Sakamoto et al,[22] 2009	24 (pancreatic mass)	Prospective	25 G	91.5%
			22 G	79.7%
			19 G trucut	51.4%
Imazu et al,[37] 2009	43 (miscellaneous)	Prospective	25 G	81%
			22 G	76%
Lee et al,[38] 2009	12 (11 pancreatic mass)	Randomised	25 G 22 G	No difference
Siddiqui et al,[39] 2009	67 (pancreatic mass)	Randomised	25 G	95%
	64 (pancreatic mass)		22 G	87%
Fabbri et al,[40] 2011	50 (pancreatic mass)	Randomised	25 G	94%
			22 G	86%
Camellini et al,[21] 2011	63 (miscellaneous)	Randomised	25 G	87%
	64 (miscellaneous)		22 G	89%
Kida et al,[27] 2011	47 (miscellaneous)	Prospective	25 G	75%
			22 G	66%
Vilmann et al,[41] 2013	135 (59 pancreas)	Prospective	22 G	89%
			25 G	90%
Song et al,[42] 2010	60 (pancreatic mass)	Randomised	19 G	84%
	57 (pancreatic mass)		22 G	78%
Songür et al,[43] 2011	35 (mediastinal lymph node)	Prospective	19 G	96%
	22 (pulmonary mass)		22 G	92%

only 65% of cases and 41% of these were not relevant for diagnosis. Immunohisto-chemistry was feasible in most cases with successful tissue procurement (91%). The overall diagnostic yield was only 52%, with mild bleeding occurring in 22% of patients and even a case of death due to abscess formation.[48]

Trucut biopsies (TCB) using 19-gauge EUS-TCB needles (Quick-Core; Cook Medical, Limerick, Ireland) are recommended when EUS-FNA turns out to be nondiagnostic, due to insufficient biopsy material (tumor cells present but of insufficient quality for definitive diagnosis or bloody specimen) as well as in cases where tissue architecture is required for diagnosis but not present (subepithelial masses, autoimmune pancreatitis, lymphoma).[49–57] It is recommended to use with caution in the esophagus, rectum, and most of the stomach. Nevertheless, the device functions with difficulties in the antrum, fundus, and duodenal bulb, where echoendoscope angulation produces sluggish advancement of the cutting sheath over the specimen tray.[51] Their lack of flexibility as well as the mechanical friction to the firing mechanism produced by the torqued echoendoscope when transduodenal biopsies are required limits their clinical usefulness. When performing transduodenal biopsies or at acute angulations, there is a need for straightening the tip of the echoendoscope, by releasing the elevator and the tip deflection; otherwise, the working channel of the echoendoscope may be damaged when the needle is fired.[2,22] Close attention should be paid to avoid traversal of the lesion and accidental puncture of adjacent structures because the needle tip advances to 20 mm on being fired.

The flexible 19-G needle (Flex 19; Boston Scientific, Natick, MA, USA), made of nitinol, could be released easily, irrespective of whether the echoendoscope tip is in a torqued or a straight position, and it did not lose its configuration, despite multiple passes.[58] In a study of 38 patients, core tissue procurement was optimal in all but 2 patients. Although on-site pathology was normal in 92% of patients, histology was required to establish a final diagnosis in 3 patients. Both the 19-G flexible needle and the latest 19-G histologic needles (ProCore; Wilson-Cook, Limerick, Ireland) have largely replaced the 19-G trucut needle for performing core biopsies. In another study, the high-definition 22-G histologic needle (ProCore; Wilson-Cook Limerick, Ireland) yielded adequate diagnostic samples with fewer passes.[59] A recent randomized study compared conventional 22-G needles and histologic 22-G needles (Pro-Core; Wilson-Cook, Limerick, Ireland) for evaluation of pancreatic masses with no differences in tumor location or size between both cohorts. The diagnostic accuracy was 100% in the case of the FNA needle and 89% in the case of ProCore needle, with the safety factor being similar for both needles.[60] Likewise, a 25-G histologic needle used in 50 consecutive patients showed a cumulative sensitivity of 83%, 91%, and 96% when cytologic analysis was performed on passes 1, 2, and 3, respectively.[61]

A pilot study of using echo-brush for sampling cystic pancreatic lesions showed superiority for diagnosis in 7 of 10 cases, compared with EUS-FNA, while some cases of intracystic bleeding were observed.[62,63] Despite initial optimism for its use, the adequacy of cytology for solid lesions was 53% and for cystic lesions of the pancreas it was only 50%. Lower results were obtained for subepithelial lesions and lymph nodes.[64]

Recently, an algorithm has been proposed to choose needles: 25-G needles for transduodenal FNA, 22-G or 25-G needles for other FNA, 19-G flexible needles for transduodenal interventions, and standard 19-G needles for interventions via other routes.[65]

Choice of Biopsy Method

The use of a stylet is considered a necessity to reduce the contamination with cells from superficial layers of the gut wall and to offer higher stability to the needle, although it enhances the rigidity of the needle apparatus when performing FNAs. Working without a stylet is possible; however, for inexperienced endosonographers the authors strongly advise using the stylet for protection of the echoendoscope channel during introduction of the needle. Several trials revealed that the diagnostic yield of malignancy, amount of blood, cellularity, contamination, and adequacy of the specimen did not differ significantly whether the stylet was used or not.[66–70] No conclusion has been drawn yet, but ESGE recommendations are that the decision on use of stylet be left to the discretion of the endosonographer performing the procedure.[2]

It is controversial whether the use of suction during EUS-FNA improves the diagnostic accuracy.[12,71–73] However, due to the capillary effect, especially in vascular lesions, the risk of bloody samples is higher.[71] In the authors' study of 52 patients with solid masses in whom 3 passes were randomized to suction or without suction, the use of suction was associated with higher diagnostic sensitivity and negative predictive values but without increasing specimen bloodiness.[74] High-pressure suction applied to a commercially available 22-G FNA needle yielded tissue samples for histologic examination in 96% of the cases and also enabled immunostaining.[75] The recommendation of ESGE is to use suction for solid masses and cystic lesions and to avoid it for lymph nodes sampling.[2]

The fanning technique, which involves sampling multiple areas within a lesion with each pass, was compared in a randomized trial with the standard to-and-fro technique. Although there was no significant difference in diagnostic accuracy between both techniques (76% vs 96%), the fanning technique facilitated a first-pass diagnosis in 85% of patients compared with less than 60% with the standard technique.[76] Using the standard technique, a survey between endosonographers reported that the accuracy for pancreatic FNA was higher than 80%. The predictive factors for higher diagnostic accuracy were more than 100 EUS-FNA case loads/year with more than 7 FNA passes being performed and the availability of rapid on-site cytopathologic evaluation or routine procurement of microcore.[77]

Initial studies indicated that the number of passes for pancreatic lesions should be 5 to 6 and for the liver or lymph nodes should be 2 to 3.[78] Whatever the type of lesion, 3 or more passes increase the diagnostic accuracy.[79] A later study observed that for pancreatic lesions no more than 7 passes (22-G needle) are necessary to obtain an accuracy of greater than 80%.[77,80] Another study observed that when performing 4 passes using the 25-G needle on solid pancreatic mass lesions, the diagnostic accuracy was similar whether an onsite cytopathologist was present or absent.[81] In a retrospective study, a mean of 2 passes with combined histology and cytology provided adequate tissue for evaluation of pancreatic masses.[31] When trucut biopsy is performed, more than 2 passes are usually necessary for improved diagnosis,[82] whereas for subepithelial lesions, 5 passes were associated with a diagnostic accuracy of 49% to 61%.[46,47]

Although the yield of cytology for cystic lesions of the pancreas is reported to be as low as 20% to 30%,[83,84] when the cysts have a solid component, performing a higher number of passes improves the diagnostic accuracy (78% vs 44%).[85] Inadequate fluid content sampling might occur in about 50% of the cases for several reasons: the cyst content might be very viscous contributing to false negative results and the limited number of passes performed (due to potential risk of infection) could lead to minimal fluid extraction and thereby yield inadequate or nondiagnostic samples.[83] The use of 19-G needles to facilitate large volume cyst aspiration or targeting the cyst wall at FNA may yield better results.

The ESGE recommends performing 3 needle passes when sampling lymph nodes and liver lesions, 5 passes when sampling solid pancreatic masses, and, a single pass when sampling pancreatic cysts due to the potential for inducing an infection.[2]

It has been demonstrated that gross visual inspection of the specimen on a slide by a trained EUS technologist or cytotechnologist was not able to predict the final cytopathologic assessment for adequacy.[86] The cytopathologic on-site rapid assessment of slides is reported to be better than monolayer prepared slides.[87] However, it is not clear if the presence of a cytopathologist ultimately improves the diagnostic accuracy.[88] Nevertheless, for suspicious lymph nodes or pancreatic masses, the diagnostic accuracy is as high as 96% with a cytopathologist versus 84% without a cytopathologist.[89] The presence of the cytopathologist also determined the need for fewer passes, lower number of inadequate samples, and higher diagnostic sensitivity.[90] Other studies showed that even the presence of a cytotechnologist can improve the interpretation for diagnostic adequacy at tissue sampling.[91,92] In the absence of a cytopathologist, the cell block evaluation of different lesions yield better diagnostic results than smear cytology (92% vs 60%).[93] For lesions accessible through the esophagus or stomach, the accuracy of EUS-TCB was equal to FNA when no on-site cytopathologist was present.[49] Specimen adequacy can be also assessed directly by the endosonographer.[94,95]

Technical Challenges During Biopsy

There exists several technical challenges during biopsy, some of which are related to designs of the needle or the echoendoscope. The rate of needle dysfunction was reported to be as high as 14% for the 22-G needle,[58,78] up to 25% for the 25-G needle,[38] and even higher for the 19-G/Trucut needle (5%–50%).[22,54,96] Even the use of 22/25 G needles was associated with technical difficulties during transduodenal punctures (24% vs 4%).[97]

Friction between the needle and the sheath is often seen during FNA via the second part of the duodenum. If this becomes problematic, it may be necessary to withdraw the echoendoscope into the stomach, adjust the length of the needle sheath as desired, and then go back through the pylorus into the duodenum and perform the FNA.

When a needle is advanced in a therapeutic channel echoendoscope, the size of the needle with its sheath covering may be unstable inside the oversized channel, resulting in insufficient needle monitoring because the unstable needle bends out of the image plane of the transducer. The solution to such a problem is to choose a needle with an appropriate sheath stabilizer (Medi-Globe GmbH, Grassau, Germany) that fits better to the size of the biopsy channel or to exchange the scope for one with a smaller channel (**Figs. 3** and **4**).

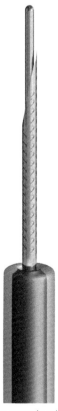

Fig. 3. Distal tip of an EUS needle with a round stylet and a tip stabilizer that increases the diameter of distal part of the sheath.

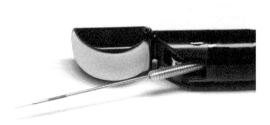

Fig. 4. The FNA needle with stabilizing tip exiting the biopsy channel of a therapeutic echoendoscope (Pentax EG 3870 UTK, Pentax Europe GmbH, Hamburg).

Detachment of the needle handle from the echoendoscope biopsy channel may occur during forceful biopsies. When this is experienced, tissue sampling must be stopped while screwing the needle handle back onto the biopsy channel. If the handle is fully detached, the biopsy needle should be retracted completely inside the protective sheath before the apparatus is engaged again to the echoendoscope.

Variable degrees of friction may be a challenge during needle advancement when performing FNA maneuvers. Tips to overcome this problem are to release the elevator after the lesion has been punctured and to reduce the angle of deflection in the echoendoscope tip. Moreover, after 1 or 2 passes, the tip of the needle may become bent, especially for 22-G and 25-G needles. When encountered, it is advisable to exchange the needle for a new one or manually (gently) straighten the tip of the needle. During the process of FNA, it may occasionally be a problem to reinsert the stylet into the needle to expel the specimen. It is suggested that needles with nitinol stylets may have less friction compared with a steel stylet.

In conclusion, there is no one technique or maneuver that is perfect for performing FNA procedures. Rather, it is a combination of minor steps and paying attention to finer details that improve the procedural outcomes.

REFERENCES

1. Polkowski M, Larghi A, Weynand B, et al. Learning techniques and complications of endoscopic ultrasound (EUS)-guided sampling in gastroenterology: European Society of Gastrointestinal Endoscopy (ESGE) Technical Guideline. Endoscopy 2012;44:190–206.
2. Savides TJ. Tricks for improving EUS-FNA accuracy and maximizing cellular yield. Gastrointest Endosc 2009;69:S130–3.
3. Gong TT, Hu DB, Zhu Q. Contrast-enhanced EUS for differential diagnosis of pancreatic mass lesions: a meta-analysi. Gastrointest Endosc 2012;75:301–9.
4. Romagnuolo J. Flow, firmness, or FNA? Is enhanced EUS fantastic or just fancy? Gastrointest Endosc 2012;76:310–2.
5. Varadarajulu S, Tamhane A, Eloubeidi MA. Yield of EUS-guided FNA of pancreatic masses in the presence or the absence of chronic pancreatitis. Gastrointest Endosc 2005;62:728–36.
6. Ranney N, Phadnis M, Trevino J, et al. Impact of biliary stents on EUS-guided FNA of pancreatic mass lesions. Gastrointest Endosc 2012;76:76–83.
7. Fisher JM, Gordon SR, Gardner TB. The impact of prior biliary stenting on the accuracy and complication rate of endoscopic ultrasound fine-needle aspiration for diagnosing pancreatic adenocarcinoma. Pancreas 2011;40:21–4.

8. Siddiqui AA, Fein M, Kowalski TE, et al. Comparison of the influence of plastic and fully covered metal biliary stents on the accuracy of EUS-FNA for the diagnosis of pancreatic cancer. Dig Dis Sci 2012;57:2438–45.

9. Ardengh JC, Lopes CV, de Lima LF, et al. Diagnosis of pancreatic tumors by endoscopic ultrasound-guided fine-needle aspiration. World J Gastroenterol 2007;13:3112–6.

10. Siddiqui AA, Brown LJ, Hong SK, et al. Relationship of pancreatic mass size and diagnostic yield of endoscopic ultrasound-guided fine needle aspiration. Dig Dis Sci 2011;56:3370–5.

11. Cheng TY, Wang HP, Jan IS, et al. Presence of intratumoral anechoic foci predicts an increased number of endoscopic ultrasound-guided fine-needle aspiration passes required for the diagnosis of pancreatic adenocarcinoma. J Gastroenterol Hepatol 2007;22:315–9.

12. Wallace MB, Kennedy T, Durkalski V, et al. Randomized controlled trial of EUS-guided fine needle aspiration techniques for the detection of malignant lymphadenopathy. Gastrointest Endosc 2001;54:441–7.

13. Bhutani MS, Saftoiu A, Chaya C, et al. Irregular echogenic foci representing coagulation necrosis: a useful but perhaps under-recognized EUS echo feature of malignant lymph node invasion. J Gastrointestin Liver Dis 2009; 18:181–4.

14. Rogart JN, Loren DE, Singu BS, et al. Cyst wall puncture and aspiration during EUS-guided fine needle aspiration may increase the diagnostic yield of mucinous cysts of the pancreas. J Clin Gastroenterol 2011;45:164–9.

15. Gupta K, Mallery S. Small-caliber endobronchial ultrasonic videoscope: successful transesophageal and transgastric FNA after failed passage of a standard ultrasonic endoscope. Gastrointest Endosc 2007;66:574–7.

16. Buxbaum JL, Eloubeidi MA. Transgastric endoscopic ultrasound (EUS) guided fine needle aspiration (FNA) in patients with esophageal narrowing using the ultrasonic bronchovideoscope. Dis Esophagus 2011;24:458–61.

17. Chatterjee S, Oppong KW. Endobronchial ultrasonic videoscope for transgastric/transesophageal fine-needle aspiration in special situations: another tool for the gastrointestinal endosonographer. Endoscopy 2012;44(Suppl 2 UCTN): E298–9.

18. Wilson JA, Hoffman B, Hawes RH, et al. EUS in patients with surgically altered upper GI anatomy. Gastrointest Endosc 2010;72:947–53.

19. Gimeno-García AZ, Elwassief A. How to improve the success of endoscopic ultrasound guided fine needle aspiration cytology in the diagnosis of pancreatic lesions. J Interv Gastroenterol 2012;2:31–6.

20. Yusuf TE, Ho S, Pavey DA, et al. Retrospective analysis of the utility of endoscopic ultrasound-guided fine-needle aspiration (EUS–FNA) in pancreatic masses, using a 22-gauge or 25-gauge needle system: a multicenter experience. Endoscopy 2009;41:445–8.

21. Camellini L, Carlinfante G, Azzolini F, et al. A randomized clinical trial comparing 22G and 25G needles in endoscopic ultrasound-guided fine-needle aspiration of solid lesions. Endoscopy 2011;43:709–15.

22. Sakamoto H, Kitano M, Komaki T, et al. Prospective comparative study of the EUS guided 25-gauge FNA needle with the 19-gauge Trucut needle and 22-gauge FNA needle in patients with solid pancreatic masses. J Gastroenterol Hepatol 2009;24:384–90.

23. Itoi T, Itokawa F, Kurihara T, et al. Experimental endoscopy: objective evaluation of EUS needles. Gastrointest Endosc 2009;69:509–16.

24. Eloubeidi MA, Jhala D, Chhieng DC, et al. Yield of endoscopic ultrasound-guided fine-needle aspiration biopsy in patients with suspected pancreatic carcinoma. Cancer 2003;99:285–92.

25. Watson RR, Binmoeller KF, Hamerski CM, et al. Yield and performance characteristics of endoscopic ultrasound-guided fine needle aspiration for diagnosing upper GI tract stromal tumors. Dig Dis Sci 2011;56:1757–62.

26. Affolter KE, Schmidt RL, Matynia AP, et al. Needle size has only a limited effect on outcomes in EUS-guided fine needle aspiration: a systematic review and meta-analysis. Dig Dis Sci 2013;58:1026–34.

27. Kida M, Araki M, Miyazawa S, et al. Comparison of diagnostic accuracy of endoscopic ultrasound-guided fine-needle aspiration with 22- and 25-gauge needles in the same patients. J Interv Gastroenterol 2011;1:102–7.

28. Eloubeidi MA, Varadarajulu S, Desai S, et al. Value of repeat endoscopic ultrasound-guided fine needle aspiration for suspected pancreatic cancer. J Gastroenterol Hepatol 2008;23:567–70.

29. Nicaud M, Hou W, Collins D, et al. The utility of repeat endoscopic ultrasound-guided fine needle aspiration for suspected pancreatic cancer. Gastroenterol Res Pract 2010;2010:268290.

30. Tadic M, Kujundzic M, Stoos-Veic T, et al. Role of repeated endoscopic ultrasound-guided fine needle aspiration in small solid pancreatic masses with previous indeterminate and negative cytological findings. Dig Dis 2008;26:377–82.

31. Möller K, Papanikolaou IS, Toermer T, et al. EUS-guided FNA of solid pancreatic masses: high yield of 2 passes with combined histologic-cytologic analysis. Gastrointest Endosc 2009;70:60–9.

32. Iglesias-Garcia J, Dominguez-Munoz E, Lozano-Leon A, et al. Impact of endoscopic ultrasound-guided fine needle biopsy for diagnosis of pancreatic masses. World J Gastroenterol 2007;13:289–93.

33. Papanikolaou IS, Adler A, Wegener K, et al. Prospective pilot evaluation of a new needle prototype for endoscopic ultrasonography-guided fine-needle aspiration: comparison of cytology and histology yield. Eur J Gastroenterol Hepatol 2008;20:342–8.

34. Yoshida S, Yamashita K, Yokozawa M, et al. Diagnostic findings of ultrasound-guided fine-needle aspiration cytology for gastrointestinal stromal tumors: proposal of a combined cytology with newly defined features and histology diagnosis. Pathol Int 2009;59:712–9.

35. Turhan N, Aydog G, Ozin Y, et al. Endoscopic ultrasonography-guided fine-needle aspiration for diagnosing upper gastrointestinal submucosal lesions: a prospective study of 50 cases. Diagn Cytopathol 2011;39:808–17.

36. Ando N, Goto H, Niwa Y, et al. The diagnosis of GI stromal tumors with EUS-guided fine needle aspiration with immunohistochemical analysis. Gastrointest Endosc 2002;55:37–43.

37. Imazu H, Uchiyama Y, Kakutani H, et al. A prospective comparison of EUS-guided FNA using 25-gauge and 22-gauge needles. Gastroenterol Res Pract 2009;2009:546390.

38. Lee JH, Stewart J, Ross WA, et al. Blinded prospective comparison of the performance of 22-gauge and 25-gauge needles in endoscopic ultrasound-guided fine needle aspiration of the pancreas and peri-pancreatic lesions. Dig Dis Sci 2009;54:2274–81.

39. Siddiqui UD, Rossi F, Rosenthal LS, et al. EUS-guided FNA of solid pancreatic masses: a prospective, randomized trial comparing 22-gauge and 25-gauge needles. Gastrointest Endosc 2009;70:1093–7.

40. Fabbri C, Polifemo AM, Luigiano C, et al. Endoscopic ultrasound-guided fine needle aspiration with 22- and 25-gauge needles in solid pancreatic masses: a prospective comparative study with randomisation of needle sequence. Dig Liver Dis 2011;43:647–52.

41. Vilmann P, Săftoiu A, Hollerbach S, et al. Multicenter randomized controlled trial comparing the performance of 22 gauge versus 25 gauge EUS-FNA needles in solid masses. Scand J Gastroenterol 2013;48:877–83.

42. Song TJ, Kim JH, Lee SS, et al. The prospective randomized, controlled trial of endoscopic ultrasound-guided fine-needle aspiration using 22G and 19G aspiration needles for solid pancreatic or peripancreatic masses. Am J Gastroenterol 2010;105:1739–45.

43. Songür N, Songür Y, Bırcan S, et al. Comparison of 19- and 22-gauge needles in EUS-guided fine needle aspiration in patients with mediastinal masses and lymph nodes. Turk J Gastroenterol 2011;22(5):472–8.

44. Itoi T, Itokawa F, Sofuni A, et al. Puncture of solid pancreatic tumors guided by endoscopic ultrasonography: a pilot study series comparing trucut and 19-gauge and 22-gauge aspiration needles. Endoscopy 2005;37:362–6.

45. Larghi A, Verna EC, Ricci R, et al. EUS-guided fine-needle tissue acquisition by using a 19-gauge needle in a selected patient population: a prospective study. Gastrointest Endosc 2011;74:504–10.

46. Mekky MA, Yamao K, Sawaki A, et al. Diagnostic utility of EUS-guided FNA in patients with gastric submucosal tumors. Gastrointest Endosc 2010;71:913–9.

47. Hoda KM, Rodriguez SA, Faigel DO. EUS-guided sampling of suspected GI stromal tumors. Gastrointest Endosc 2009;69(7):1218–23.

48. Eckardt AJ, Adler A, Gomes EM, et al. Endosonographic large-bore biopsy of gastric subepithelial tumors: a prospective multicenter study. Eur J Gastroenterol Hepatol 2012;24:1135–44.

49. Storch I, Jorda M, Thurer R, et al. Advantage of EUS Trucut biopsy combined with fine-needle aspiration without immediate on-site cytopathologic examination. Gastrointest Endosc 2006;64:505–11.

50. Săftoiu A, Vilmann P, Guldhammer Skov B, et al. Endoscopic ultrasound (EUS)-guided Trucut biopsy adds significant information to EUS-guided fine-needleaspiration in selected patients: a prospective study. Scand J Gastroenterol 2007; 42:117–25.

51. Levy MJ, Wiersema MJ. EUS-guided Trucut biopsy. Gastrointest Endosc 2005; 62:417–26.

52. DeWitt J, Emerson RE, Sherman S, et al. Endoscopic ultrasound-guided Trucut biopsy of gastrointestinal mesenchymal tumor. Surg Endosc 2011;25: 2192–202.

53. Larghi A, Verna EC, Stavropoulos SN, et al. EUS-guided trucut needle biopsies in patients with solid pancreatic masses: a prospective study. Gastrointest Endosc 2004;59:185–90.

54. Fernández-Esparrach G, Sendino O, Solé M, et al. Endoscopic ultrasound-guided fine-needle aspiration and trucut biopsy in the diagnosis of gastric stromal tumors: a randomized crossover study. Endoscopy 2010;42:292–9.

55. Storch I, Shah M, Thurer R, et al. Endoscopic ultrasound-guided fine-needle aspiration and Trucut biopsy in thoracic lesions: when tissue is the issue. Surg Endosc 2008;22(1):86–90.

56. Polkowski M, Gerke W, Jarosz D, et al. Diagnostic yield and safety of endoscopic ultrasound-guided trucut [corrected] biopsy in patients with gastric submucosal tumors: a prospective study. Endoscopy 2009;41:329–34.

57. Wahnschaffe U, Ullrich R, Mayerle J, et al. EUS-guided Trucut needle biopsies as first-line diagnostic method for patients with intestinal or extraintestinal mass lesions. Surg Endosc 2009;23:2351–5.

58. Varadarajulu S, Bang JY, Hebert-Magee S. Assessment of the technical performance of the flexible 19-gauge EUS-FNA needle. Gastrointest Endosc 2012;76:336–43.

59. Witt BL, Adler DG, Hilden K, et al. A comparative needle study: EUS-FNA procedures using the HD ProCore™ and EchoTip® 22-gauge needle types. Diagn Cytopathol, in press.

60. Bang JY, Hebert-Magee S, Trevino J, et al. Randomized trial comparing the 22-gauge aspiration and 22-gauge biopsy needles for EUS-guided sampling of solid pancreatic mass lesions. Gastrointest Endosc 2012;76:321–7.

61. Iwashita T, Nakai Y, Samarasena JB, et al. High single-pass diagnostic yield of a new 25-gauge core biopsy needle for EUS-guided FNA biopsy in solid pancreatic lesions. Gastrointest Endosc 2013;77:909–15.

62. Al-Haddad M, Raimondo M, Woodward T, et al. Safety and efficacy of cytology brushings versus standard FNA in evaluating cystic lesions of the pancreas: a pilot study. Gastrointest Endosc 2007;65:894–8.

63. Al-Haddad M, Gill KR, Raimondo M, et al. Safety and efficacy of cytology brushings versus standard fine-needle aspiration in evaluating cystic pancreatic lesions: a controlled study. Endoscopy 2010;42:127–32.

64. Bruno M, Bosco M, Carucci P, et al. Preliminary experience with a new cytology brush in EUS-guided FNA. Gastrointest Endosc 2009;70:1220–4.

65. Bang JY, Ramesh J, Trevino J, et al. Objective assessment of an algorithmic approach to EUS-guided FNA and interventions. Gastrointest Endosc 2013;77:739–44.

66. Rastogi A, Wani S, Gupta N, et al. A prospective, single-blind, randomized, controlled trial of EUS-guided FNA with and without a stylet. Gastrointest Endosc 2011;74:58–64.

67. Sahai AV, Paquin SC, Gariépy G. A prospective comparison of endoscopic ultrasound-guided fine needle aspiration results obtained in the same lesion, with and without the needle stylet. Endoscopy 2010;42:900–3.

68. Wani S, Early D, Kunkel J, et al. Diagnostic yield of malignancy during EUS-guided FNA of solid lesions with and without a stylet: a prospective, single blind, randomized, controlled trial. Gastrointest Endosc 2012;76:328–35.

69. Gimeno-García AZ, Paquin SC, Gariépy G, et al. Comparison of endoscopic ultrasonography-guided fine-needle aspiration cytology results with and without the stylet in 3364 cases. Dig Endosc 2012;25:303–7.

70. Wani S, Gupta N, Gaddam S, et al. A comparative study of endoscopic ultrasound guided fine needle aspiration with and without a stylet. Dig Dis Sci 2011;56:2409–14.

71. Lee JK, Choi JH, Lee KH, et al. A prospective, comparative trial to optimize sampling techniques in EUS-guided FNA of solid pancreatic masses. Gastrointest Endosc 2013;77:745–51.

72. Thomson HD. Thin needle aspiration biopsy. Acta Cytol 1982;26:262–3.

73. Bhutani MS, Suryaprasad S, Moezzi J, et al. Improved technique for performing endoscopic ultrasound guided fine needle aspiration of lymph nodes. Endoscopy 1999;31:550–3.

74. Puri R, Vilmann P, Săftoiu A, et al. Randomized controlled trial of endoscopic ultrasound-guided fine-needle sampling with or without suction for better cytological diagnosis. Scand J Gastroenterol 2009;44:499–504.

75. Larghi A, Noffsinger A, Dye CE, et al. EUS-guided fine needle tissue acquisition by using high negative pressure suction for the evaluation of solid masses: a pilot study. Gastrointest Endosc 2005;62:768–74.
76. Bang JY, Magee SH, Ramesh J, et al. Randomized trial comparing fanning with standard technique for endoscopic ultrasound-guided fine-needle aspiration of solid pancreatic mass lesions. Endoscopy 2013;45:445–50.
77. Dumonceau JM, Koessler T, van Hooft JE, et al. Endoscopic ultrasonography-guided fine needle aspiration: relatively low sensitivity in the endosonographer population. World J Gastroenterol 2012;18:2357–63.
78. Erickson RA, Sayage-Rabie L, Beissner RS. Factors predicting the number of EUS-guided fine-needle passes for diagnosis of pancreatic malignancies. Gastrointest Endosc 2000;51:184–90.
79. Rong L, Kida M, Yamauchi H, et al. Factors affecting the diagnostic accuracy of endoscopic ultrasonography-guided fine-needle aspiration (EUS-FNA) for upper gastrointestinal submucosal or extraluminal solid mass lesions. Dig Endosc 2012;24:358–63.
80. LeBlanc JK, Ciaccia D, Al-Assi MT, et al. Optimal number of EUS-guided fine needle passes needed to obtain a correct diagnosis. Gastrointest Endosc 2004;59:475–81.
81. Suzuki R, Irisawa A, Bhutani MS, et al. Prospective evaluation of the optimal number of 25-gauge needle passes for endoscopic ultrasound-guided fine-needle aspiration biopsy of solid pancreatic lesions in the absence of an onsite cytopathologist. Dig Endosc 2012;24:452–6.
82. Thomas T, Kaye PV, Ragunath K, et al. Efficacy, safety, and predictive factors for a positive yield of EUS-guided Trucut biopsy: a large tertiary referral center experience. Am J Gastroenterol 2009;104:584–91.
83. de Jong K, Poley JW, van Hooft JE, et al. Endoscopic ultrasound-guided fine-needle aspiration of pancreatic cystic lesions provides inadequate material for cytology and laboratory analysis: initial results from a prospective study. Endoscopy 2011;43:585–90.
84. Maire F, Couvelard A, Hammel P, et al. Intraductal papillary mucinous tumors of the pancreas: the preoperative value of cytologic and histopathologic diagnosis. Gastrointest Endosc 2003;58:701–6.
85. Lim LG, Lakhtakia S, Ang TL, et al. Factors determining diagnostic yield of endoscopic ultrasound guided fine-needle aspiration for pancreatic cystic lesions: a multicentre Asian study. Dig Dis Sci 2013;58:1751–7.
86. Nguyen YP, Maple JT, Zhang Q, et al. Reliability of gross visual assessment of specimen adequacy during EUS-guided FNA of pancreatic masses. Gastrointest Endosc 2009;69:1264–70.
87. LeBlanc JK, Emerson RE, Dewitt J, et al. A prospective study comparing rapid assessment of smears and ThinPrep for endoscopic ultrasound-guided fine-needle aspirates. Endoscopy 2010;42:389–94.
88. Eloubeidi MA, Tamhane A, Jhala N, et al. Agreement between rapid onsite and final cytologic interpretations of EUS-guided FNA specimens: implications for the endosonographer and patient management. Am J Gastroenterol 2006; 101:2841–7.
89. Cleveland P, Gill KR, Coe SG, et al. An evaluation of risk factors for inadequate cytology in EUS-guided FNA of pancreatic tumors and lymph nodes. Gastrointest Endosc 2010;71:1194–9.
90. Iglesias-Garcia J, Dominguez-Munoz JE, Abdulkader I, et al. Influence of on-site cytopathology evaluation on the diagnostic accuracy of endoscopic

ultrasound-guided fine needle aspiration (EUS-FNA) of solid pancreatic masses. Am J Gastroenterol 2011;106:1705–10.

91. Alsohaibani F, Girgis S, Sandha GS. Does onsite cytotechnology evaluation improve the accuracy of endoscopic ultrasound-guided fine-needle aspiration biopsy? Can J Gastroenterol 2009;23:26–30.
92. Turner BG, Cizginer S, Agarwal D, et al. Diagnosis of pancreatic neoplasia with EUS and FNA: a report of accuracy. Gastrointest Endosc 2010;71:91–8.
93. Noda Y, Fujita N, Kobayashi G, et al. Diagnostic efficacy of the cell block method in comparison with smear cytology of tissue samples obtained by endoscopic ultrasound-guided fine-needle aspiration. J Gastroenterol 2010;45: 868–75.
94. Savoy AD, Raimondo M, Woodward TA, et al. Can endosonographers evaluate on-site cytologic adequacy? A comparison with cytotechnologists. Gastrointest Endosc 2007;65:953–7.
95. Hikichi T, Irisawa A, Bhutani MS, et al. Endoscopic ultrasound-guided fine-needle aspiration of solid pancreatic masses with rapid on-site cytological evaluation by endosonographers without attendance of cytopathologists. J Gastroenterol 2009;44:322–8.
96. Varadarajulu S, Fraig M, Schmulewitz N, et al. Comparison of EUS-guided 19-gauge Trucut needle biopsy with EUS-guided fine-needle aspiration. Endoscopy 2004;36:397–401.
97. Varadarajulu S, Blakely J, Latif SU, et al. Quality assessment of current EUS-FNA assembly performance: adequate for use or opportunity for improvement? Gastrointest Endosc 2011;73:AB174–5.

Pitfalls in EUS FNA

Larissa L. Fujii, MD*, Michael J. Levy, MD

KEYWORDS

- Endosonography • Fine-needle aspiration • Cytopathology • Diagnostic yield
- Limitation

KEY POINTS

- Endoscopic ultrasound (EUS)-guided fine-needle aspiration (FNA) should be performed only if the results will potentially impact patient care as determined by the patients' multi-disciplinary team.
- Direct communication between the endosonographer and cytotechnologist and cytopathologist is key to optimize the specimen adequacy and diagnostic accuracy.
- False-negative cytology most commonly results from sampling error caused by inaccurate sampling by the endosonographer, suboptimal characteristics of the target lesion, or misinterpretation of on-site cytology review.
- The presence of chronic pancreatitis negatively impacts both EUS imaging and FNA cytologic interpretation, thereby decreasing the diagnostic yield of EUS FNA.

INTRODUCTION

Since the introduction of endoscopic ultrasound (EUS)-guided fine-needle aspiration (FNA) in the early 1990s, the technique has emerged as a method of choice for tissue acquisition in the diagnosis of a broad spectrum of intra-abdominal and intrathoracic malignancies.[1,2] Virtually any lesion or organ that lies in close vicinity to the gastrointestinal (GI) tract can be accessed with an FNA needle. However, as for any procedure, EUS FNA has its limitations. These pitfalls, which can occur before, during, or after the procedure, are important to understand in order to optimize the accuracy, efficiency, and safety of the examination.

PREPROCEDURAL PITFALLS
Failure to Establish Clinical and Procedural Goals

EUS FNA typically represents only one component of an often-broad diagnostic strategy. A clear understanding of the clinical and procedural goals is necessary to guide

Disclosures: The authors have nothing to disclose.
Division of Gastroenterology and Hepatology, Mayo Clinic, 200 1st Street Southwest, Rochester, MN 55905, USA
* Corresponding author.
E-mail address: fujii.larissa@mayo.edu

Gastrointest Endoscopy Clin N Am 24 (2014) 125–142
http://dx.doi.org/10.1016/j.giec.2013.08.003
1052-5157/14/$ – see front matter © 2014 Elsevier Inc. All rights reserved.

patient care decisions. The goals must be carefully considered, based on sound clinical judgment, and fully discussed with patients and families. The goals help guide procedural planning, allow targeting of FNA sites, clarify potential anatomic obstacles, and may indicate a more accurate, cost-effective, or safer alternative to EUS FNA.

The clinical and procedural goals and decision whether to perform EUS FNA should be made in a multidisciplinary manner to resolve controversies that often exist between and within subspecialties regarding the role of EUS FNA. The procedure should only be considered if the results would impact patient management.[3] For instance, in patients with obstructive jaundice who have a characteristic-appearing resectable pancreatic carcinoma on computed tomography (CT) and EUS, the need for a preoperative tissue diagnosis is debated. In this setting, it is imperative to understand the views of the surgeon, oncologist, and pancreatologist regarding the role of FNA. Some argue against FNA because an alternate diagnosis is seldom discovered because of the false-negative rate of FNA and because of the risk of tumor seeding or pancreatitis that may complicate or delay surgery. The potential advantages and arguments for FNA include the need for a tissue diagnosis when administering neoadjuvant therapy, detection of less common pancreatic neoplasms (eg, neuroendocrine tumors, lymphoma, or metastasis) or a benign process (eg, autoimmune pancreatitis) that would be managed differently, and to assist in patient counseling. Regardless of the approach in your institution, the views of the patients and the medical team must be considered to establish the procedural goals in order to optimize patient care and minimize legal exposure.

Failure to Obtain a Thorough Informed Consent

Many issues must be addressed during the informed-consent process, including an explanation of the procedure and the potential benefits, risks, and alternatives. To help ensure the procedural goals are met and to avoid repeat examinations, the authors suggest that the consent process also include a discussion of specific pitfalls, most notably the potential for a false-negative EUS FNA interpretation. As discussed later, a negative test result may lead to diagnostic confusion and uncertainty as to whether the negative finding represents a true- or false-negative result. This occurrence often necessitates repeat procedures (eg, EUS, percutaneous, or surgical) to obtain a tissue diagnosis and complicates patient counseling. Patients should also be informed of the potential need for alternate biopsy devices (eg, larger- or smaller-caliber standard FNA needles or core biopsy needles). Their use may be necessary following the initial inconclusive biopsy results and/or to obtain specimens that allow histologic examination (eg, subepithelial lesions, lymphoma, and autoimmune pancreatitis). Although some consider their use inherent to the consent process, this is not the case in all institutions given the potential impact on cost and safety. Also, there are non-FNA interventions that may directly or indirectly affect FNA results, including the need for cystic fluid analysis, celiac plexus neurolysis (CPN) in the case of confirmed metastatic pancreatic cancer, or EUS-guided ductal access. Again, although some interventions may be considered implied, the authors favor specific discussion during the informed-consent process.

Failure to Review Noninvasive Imaging and Laboratory Test Results

EUS examinations are often facilitated by the results of noninvasive imaging, including transabdominal ultrasound, CT, and magnetic resonance imaging/cholangiopancreatography and relevant laboratory test results. The findings may be used to determine the need for EUS, guide procedural planning, allow targeting of FNAs, complement EUS staging, clarify potential anatomic obstacles, or indicate a preferred alternative route for tissue acquisition. For instance, the detection of right hepatic lobe metastasis would indicate a patient who may be better served by percutaneous FNA to avoid the expense and risk associated with EUS and the accompanying sedation. However, even in this setting, EUS may be performed in a cost-effective manner if therapeutic intervention is also planned (eg, CPN). A review of the clinical goals and findings of noninvasive imaging and laboratory results can help guide these management decisions. Therefore, it is essential to obtain and interpret relevant laboratory results and imaging that should also be readily available for comparison during the EUS examination.

Insufficient Training or Experience

The experience and skill of an endosonographer are critical to the success of EUS imaging and guided biopsy. The ability to locate sites of pathology and to distinguish them from normal structures is equally important as the requisite skills to perform FNA. In one study, endosonographer experience was the only factor on multivariate analysis that predicted the EUS FNA diagnostic accuracy, which measured 33% and 91% for initial versus later experience, respectively.[4] The current guidelines from the American Society for Gastrointestinal Endoscopy (ASGE) requires a minimum of 150 supervised EUS procedures and 50 supervised EUS FNA (25 pancreatic and 25 nonpancreatic masses each) before assessing competency.[5] These thresholds are supported by the findings of a study demonstrating a significant increase in EUS FNA diagnostic sensitivity of pancreatic cancers after 30 cases.[6] The learning curve has been shown to continue well after training, with subsequent improvement in an endosonographer's diagnostic accuracy and examination efficiency.[7] The ASGE-recommended procedural volumes are advocated by many and are appropriate in certain practice settings. However, the authors regard the suggested minimum EUS volumes and level of training as far insufficient to permit independent practice within a tertiary referral center.

Please refer to **Box 1** for a summary of some of the preprocedural pitfalls that may be encountered.

INTRAPROCEDURAL PITFALLS
Inability to Access the Target Lesion

EUS FNA cannot be performed when the target lesion is inaccessible, which may be the situation for patients with altered anatomy. For instance, altered anatomy limits visualization and access to pancreaticobiliary lesions, particularly after Roux-en-Y surgery.[8] Among all 13 patients with Roux-en-Y anatomy in this study, imaging of the pancreatic head and bile duct was impaired because of the inability to reach the proximal duodenum. Similarly, the success of pancreaticobiliary imaging with gastric bypass, Billroth II, or Puestow anatomy was only 14%, 48%, and 50%, respectively. The main limitations were the inability to intubate the afferent limb or proximal small bowel and the presence of intervening small bowel gas. The investigators reported successful pancreaticobiliary EUS in most of the patients following a Billroth I, Whipple, Nissen fundoplication, or esophagectomy. In the authors' practice, although they are mindful to the potential impact of surgically altered anatomy, they do not view this as a contraindication to EUS because the target lesion can often be accessed from various sites within the bowel. As shown by other investigators, EUS can be technically successful for most patients undergoing pancreatic EUS after Billroth II gastrectomy.[9] In addition, the clinical goals can often be achieved through the detection and biopsy of other known or previously unappreciated sites of pathologic disease, thereby obviating the biopsy of nonaccessible sites.

Box 1
Preprocedural pitfalls of EUS FNA

Failure to establish procedural goals

- Failure to have a discussion with the multidisciplinary team to determine utility and role of EUS FNA
- Performing EUS FNA in patients when the results would not impact management
- Failure to establish the role of FNA for resectable versus unresectable malignancies
- Neglecting to perform EUS FNA for diagnostic confirmation before chemoradiation

Failure to obtain a thorough informed consent

- Lack or inadequate discussion of the procedure, potential benefits, risks, and alternatives
- Not discussing the potential for a false-negative EUS FNA test result and resulting implications
- Not discussing the potential need and risks of alternative EUS biopsy devices
- Not discussing other non-FNA interventions that may take place during the procedure

Failure to obtain and/or review noninvasive imaging and laboratory tests

- Unable to recognize features that may complicate the procedure (eg, altered anatomy)
- Failure to recognize distant sites of disease that may obviate the biopsy of the primary tumor or indicate a preferred alternative route for tissue acquisition
- Failure to recognize inadequate drainage of biliary obstruction before EUS FNA of a liver lesion
- Failure to recognize complementary staging information

Failure to recognize contraindications

- Presence of a contraindication (coagulopathy, antiplatelet or antithrombotic medication, significant comorbid illness, and so forth) resulting in adverse event or procedure cancellation

Inappropriate selection of adequate sedation

- Inadequate sedation leading to an incomplete examination or patient movement that risks a difficult/inadequate FNA

Endosonographer inexperience

- Inability to differentiate normal anatomy from pathology (eg, tumor vs inflammation)
- Unable to recognize characteristic EUS imaging features that may improperly alter the use of FNA
- Limited understanding of the anatomy
- Skilled use of the radial but not linear echoendoscope
- Lack of knowledge regarding FNA and other biopsy devices needles
- Lack of endoscopic or FNA technical skills (eg, unable to adjust for needle bending)
- Inability to visualize the tip of the needle during sampling
- Insufficient training (mentorship or volume) that limits continued learning after formal training

Lesions may also be inaccessible because of a luminal obstruction that prohibits the passage of the echoendoscope because of the presence of intervening structures within the needle path (eg, bile or pancreatic ducts or blood vessels), retained luminal contents (eg, food) that impair acoustic coupling and/or increase the procedural risk (eg, local infection or airway aspiration), or the presence of excessive air in the visual field (eg, intervening bowel or airway). In additions lesions may be considered inaccessible if they are located beyond the range of EUS imaging or needle access (eg, portions of the right hepatic lobe) or when lying deep to a primary luminal tumor (eg, lymph nodes) because of the risk of a false-positive FNA secondary to the resulting needle path.[10]

Failure to Obtain FNAs in an Algorithmic Manner

It is important to prioritize the sequence of FNA sites using an algorithmic approach.[11] The goal of EUS FNA is not only to establish a tissue diagnosis but also to enhance the staging accuracy over EUS imaging alone. These biopsies and resulting information must be acquired in a safe and efficient manner. These goals are most clearly met when prioritizing the sequence of FNAs to initial biopsy sites that most significantly impact tumor stage and patient management. Only when initial biopsies are nondiagnostic should sites that offer less prognostic information or greater risk be sampled. One should also consider the number of biopsies necessary to establish the diagnosis, which varies among sites.[12-14] For instance, when considering these issues (prognostic information vs safety) in patients with a suspected pancreatic carcinoma, the authors' approach is to obtain FNAs from sites suspected of containing metastasis using the following sequence: (1) malignant-appearing distant lymph nodes, (2) omental deposits or ascitic fluid, (3) malignant-appearing liver mass, and (4) a malignant-appearing local lymph node. Only when these sites are benign appearing and not sampled or when specimens are interpreted as benign do they perform FNA of the pancreatic mass. This approach establishes the diagnosis without the need for pancreatic FNAs in 10% to 20% of patients and avoids the risks associated with pancreatic biopsy.[13,15-19] This method of biopsy also provides the greatest impact on staging and patient care.

Lesion Characteristics that Contribute to a Difficult FNA

Echoendoscope position

The target lesion site and, therefore, location of the echoendoscope within the GI tract has some bearing on the technical success and sample adequacy of EUS FNA. For instance, transesophageal FNA is facilitated by the straight course of the esophagus, which allows less deflection of the echoendoscope and needle, thereby imparting less resistance to needle advancement. In addition, the narrow lumen of the esophagus serves to help constrain the echoendoscope and diminishes the tendency for echoendoscope recoil on needle advancement. The larger luminal diameter and somewhat tortuous shape of the stomach and rectum leads to some difficulty during EUS-guided biopsy. The technical challenges are most pronounced when obtaining biopsies from the gastric fundus and the second portion of the duodenum where severe angulation can even prohibit advance of the needle through the echoendoscope and risk instrument damage. These limitations are most pronounced when using larger-caliber or trucut biopsy needles.

EUS FNA success is optimized by several technical considerations, such as retracting and straightening the echoendoscope, and by reducing echoendoscope angulation and elevator use.[20,21] Although these steps help minimize the sluggish advancement of the biopsy device, the short-scope position predisposes to inadvertent scope retraction from the duodenum. The tendency for instrument recoil within a large-diameter lumen is minimized by removing air from the lumen, by using the up-down ratchet to provide firm apposition of the transducer to the bowel wall, and with quick needle advancement.[11,21] When severe angulation prohibits full needle insertion within the echoendoscope, the needle can usually be safely advanced with tip deflection in the opposite direction. When not successful, it may be necessary to initially advance the needle while positioned in the stomach before proceeding to the duodenum. Care must be taken to use proper needle adaptor spacing to avoid overly advancing the needle, which may injure the bowel wall during echoendoscope repositioning.

Lesion size

The size of the target lesion may also influence FNA results, although evidence is inconsistent. Some have shown that smaller lesions are more challenging to biopsy and yield a lower diagnostic yield.[22] Alternatively, several studies failed to show that the lesion size significantly altered the FNA sample adequacy.[23–27] In fact, some data suggest that FNA of larger lesions that contain areas of necrosis is associated with lower diagnostic sensitivity. Therefore, the practice of targeting the periphery of a large lesion or fanning the needle tip in multiple trajectories to increase the sample volume may increase the diagnostic yield of FNA.[11,28,29]

Lesion consistency

The consistency of a lesion also contributes to the ease of needle puncture. For instance, indurated lesions, such as pancreatic adenocarcinomas that contain a dense desmoplastic reaction and fibrosis, are harder lesions and more difficult to perform FNA. Such lesions may bend or dull the needle, necessitating needle straightening between passes or the use of additional needles. FNA of indurated lesions is facilitated by echoendoscope tip deflection into the luminal wall, by rapid and more forceful needle advancement, and the use of smaller-caliber needles.[11,28] Desmoplastic tumors also are challenging for the cytopathologist because neoplastic cells typically lie within abundant amounts of collagen and necrosis and because of the typical paucicellular specimen. Therefore, because the FNA needle preferentially gathers cells that detach easily, benign cells often predominant within the specimen.[30] Additional needle passes are often required to aid the cytopathology review.

Incorrect Specimen Handling and Preparation

Although practice varies among institutions, the EUS FNA specimen is typically expelled from the needle using an air-filled syringe or by advancing the stylet. A portion of the specimen is expelled onto a prelabeled glass slide, and the remaining material is placed in a liquid-based cytology container for cell-block preparation. This process should be timely to avoid clotting, which may disrupt the process of smearing on the slide. The technologist should be trained in proper labeling, sample distribution onto slides versus liquid-based cytology, and appropriate smearing, fixation, and staining. Overly thick smears can disrupt aggregates of benign cells that may falsely appear malignant because of the loss of cell cohesion.[30] Drying before fixation may cause artifactual nuclear enlargement, which can mask the difference between reactive lymphoid tissue and lymphoma.[30] Care must also be taken to distribute the specimen in a manner consistent with the goals of the practice. For instance, in the authors' practice, a larger portion of the specimen is allocated for immediate review to enhance the in-room diagnostic sensitivity. The authors think that this practice more directly and accurately guides the number of FNAs obtained and may improve overall diagnostic accuracy. The authors typically continue sampling until an in-room diagnosis is achieved. This approach provides less material for cell blocks and subsequent review. On the contrary, some practices preferentially allocate more of the specimen for cell block review, which may optimize the final review but negatively impacts in-room interpretation.

Poor Endosonographer and Cytopathologist Communication

Direct communication between the endosonographer and cytopathologist/cytotechnician is essential. The endosonographer should relay pertinent clinical, radiographic, and laboratory information concerning patients. For instance, awareness of the use of prior treatment is important because nuclear atypia resulting from chemoradiation may be misinterpreted as malignancy.[30] Similarly, knowledge of prior cancers or inflammatory processes may call attention to unsuspected or rare pathologies and focus the pathology review. The site of the GI tract that the FNA needle traverses, as well as intervening tissues, should be conveyed to help eliminate the risk of misinterpreting contaminating elements. The lesion from which tissue is acquired also helps the cytopathologist develop a more focused differential for accurate diagnosis.

Incorrect or Misleading On-site Cytopathology Review

Rapid on-site evaluation (ROSE) of cytologic samples is used to determine specimen adequacy and to guide the need for further FNA to establish a diagnosis or determine a need for ancillary testing.[31] A recent meta-analysis found that ROSE was associated with improved FNA sample adequacy rates in centers with an initially low adequacy rate (<90%) but was not associated with increased diagnostic yield.[32] The adequacy rates were superior for on-site cytopathologists as compared with cytotechnologists or residents. Cytopathologist and cytotechnologist experience critically impacts the diagnostic yield of EUS FNA. Formal cytotechnology training has been shown to improve the diagnostic accuracy and decrease the number of FNA passes required to achieve a diagnosis.[33] Such training is necessary to allow accurate interpretation of specimens that are often paucicellular and routinely include contaminated material from the GI epithelium, intervening tissues, and from nondiagnostic regions of the target lesion.[28,31] Unfortunately, the use of cytopathologists for ROSE is hampered by their other clinical demands and poor reimbursement.[34] Therefore, most institutions rely on cytotechnologists and residents to assess the FNA specimens in the EUS suite, with real-time telecytology available in few centers.[35] Despite the potential utility of ROSE, the risk of inaccurate in-room interpretation remains, sometimes necessitating repeat EUS. Partly for this reason, there has been a migration in the expectations and role of the on-site cytopathology review. Historically in the authors' center and still true in some institutions, the goal of the on-site review was solely to determine the cellularity and sample adequacy. The authors consider this no longer to be an acceptable threshold because a specimen may contain a large quantity of the representative organ or tissue and be deemed an adequate sample but fail to contain the material necessary to establish a diagnosis. The authors instead work to achieve a diagnosis instead of simply obtaining a cellular or representative sample.

Incorrect or Misleading Final Cytopathology Review

In a recent meta-analysis of 41 studies, the pooled sensitivity and specificity of EUS FNA of solid pancreatic masses were 86.8% (95% confidence interval [CI] 85.5–87.9) and 95.8% (95% CI 94.6–96.7), respectively.[36] The diagnostic accuracy of EUS FNA for mediastinal lymph nodes was similar,[37] but the sensitivity for pancreatic cystic neoplasms was much lower at 54% (95% CI 49–59).[38] The diagnostic yield of EUS FNA in most centers is likely lower than reported in the literature.[39] In a study polling an international group of endosonographers, only a third of the respondents reported a sensitivity greater than 80% for solid masses. It was thought that greater sensitivity was achieved when obtaining more than 7 FNA passes, with the use of ROSE, for high procedural volumes and with routine use of paraffin-embedded cell blocks.

False-negative diagnoses, or low diagnostic sensitivity, are common and estimated to occur in 4% to 45% of solid pancreatic masses,[40–42] 21% to 53% of pancreatic cystic neoplasms,[42,43] 6% to 14% of lymph nodes,[44,45] and 0% to 17% of biliary strictures with benign cytology.[46–48] The most common cause of a false-negative examination is sampling error with insufficient material presented to the cytopathologist. Sample inadequacy may be attributed to the endosonographer (eg, errors in image recognition or poorly targeted biopsy), the target lesion (eg, low tumor density or well differentiated tumors), or on-site cytology review (eg, misinterpretation), and often the presence of more than one variable.[30,40] In one study, 19 patients (19%) with negative or atypical cytology were confirmed by surgery to have a pancreatic adenocarcinoma (n = 8), neuroendocrine tumor (n = 3), or pancreatic cystic neoplasm (n = 8, 2 with associated adenocarcinoma).[42] Among these 19 discrepant cases, 89% were attributed to sampling error versus 11% resulting from cytopathology misinterpretation. Sampling error was more commonly seen in cystic lesions than solid pancreatic masses (33% and 12%, respectively, $P<.05$). Despite the higher false-negative rate seen in cystic pancreatic tumors (CPT), the use of EUS FNA has been shown to incrementally increase the diagnostic yield over radiologic imaging.[49] The diagnostic challenge of CPT highlights the importance of using patients' clinical presentation, serial radiographic studies, FNA cytology, and ancillary studies in combination to establish a diagnosis. Relying solely on FNA results in the case of a false-negative test will lead to delayed and/or improper patient care and inappropriate reassurance to the patients, all negatively impacting patient outcomes.

Similarly, false-positive (ie, low diagnostic specificity) EUS FNA results may also be attributed to sampling error and cytopathologist misinterpretation. One study identified 377 patients with EUS FNA cytology interpreted as positive or suspicious for malignancy who had a gold standard diagnosis based on direct surgical resection without prior neoadjuvant therapy.[10] The false-positive rate was 20 out of 377 (5.3%) and increased to 27 out of 377 (7.2%) when false-suspicious cases were included. Based on root cause analysis and cytopathologist blind consensus re-review of all specimens, 50% of the errors were attributed to the endosonographer (eg, sampling error) or procedure itself (eg, translocated cell contamination) and 50% were attributed to cytopathologist interpretive error.[10] Most of the false-positive results occurred in nonpancreatic samples, including FNA of periesophageal or perirectal lymph nodes in the setting of luminal malignancy. Contamination by GI tract epithelial cells and tumor cells within the luminal fluid contributed to the higher rates of false-positive specimens in the setting of luminal cancers. This connection was highlighted in a study that collected the luminal fluid present within the suction channel of the echoendoscope before and after EUS FNA.[50] Luminal fluid–positive cytology from these specimens was found in 48% of patients with luminal cancer, 10% of patients with extraluminal cancer, and no patient with nonmalignant disease. A separate study attributed 3 false-positive EUS FNA results to endometriosis, a duodenal diverticulum with smooth muscle hyperplasia, and a normal pancreas possibly with heterotopic pancreatic tissue within the duodenal mucosa.[51] A false-positive FNA result may substantially impair patient care and outcomes. For instance, falsely interpreting a benign process as malignant may lead to inappropriate use of chemoradiation or surgical resection. In addition, a false-positive FNA result may lead to incorrect upstaging of an existing neoplasia leading to an incorrect designation of unresectability and incurability, leading one to forego potentially life-saving intervention.

Diagnostic Challenges by Site

Chronic pancreatitis (CP) is well known to decrease the diagnostic accuracy of EUS FNA. In one report, the sensitivity of diagnosing a pancreatic malignancy decreased from 89% in patients with a normal pancreas to 54% in patients with CP.[52] Another study reported a diagnostic sensitivity of 91.3% versus 73.9% in patients without and with CP, respectively.[53] The investigators noted that the sensitivity was improved by increasing the number of FNA passes. The presence of CP negatively impacts both EUS imaging and FNA cytologic interpretation. It may be difficult to rely on imaging to distinguish a malignant mass from masslike (ie, tumefactive) CP. This difficulty is most notable in the presence of significant lobularity, focal pancreatitis, or calcification with postacoustic shadowing or coexisting acute pancreatitis.[28,53] Cytologic interpretation is impaired when finding a polymorphous cell population and the presence of desmoplasia and inflammatory epithelial changes that are common to both CP and pancreatic adenocarcinoma.[31,54]

Cytology provides a low sensitivity for diagnosing CPT because of the typically sparse number of cysts lining epithelial cells and contaminating protein, blood, and inflammatory cells.[30,38] In addition, the presence of translocated duodenal or gastric luminal epithelial cells may lead to a false diagnosis of a mucinous CPT.[31] The accuracy of EUS FNA for diagnosing CPT is improved when sampling a solid component if present.[55] Although cyst wall puncture and brushing during EUS FNA may increase the diagnosis of intracellular mucin in CPT, the practice has not been widely practiced because of the potential for major complications, including death.[56–58] Similarly, EUS-guided trucut biopsy of the cyst wall or solid component may provide an otherwise unattainable diagnosis.[21] However, its use is limited given the design flaws and difficult use.

Pancreatic neuroendocrine tumors (PNET) can be diagnosed by EUS FNA in 83% to 100% of patients.[59–61] Despite the high diagnostic yield, PNET can display a variety of cytologic features, which often complicates the diagnosis.[62] Pancreatic splenosis and intrapancreatic lymph nodes are both benign conditions that mimic PNET on EUS and other radiographic studies as well as by EUS FNA.[63–65] CP may also cytologically mimic PNET, with acinar loss and fibrosis resulting in islet cell aggregation or hyperplasia.[66] In addition, clear-cell PNET have a cytologic appearance similar to renal cell carcinoma or solid pseudopapillary tumors. Finally, acinar cell tumors are often cytologically confused with PNET.[67,68]

Failure to Use Ancillary Techniques

Ancillary pathology tests provide an important adjunct to cytologic examination, particularly for indeterminate lesions. Ancillary studies require adequate tissue sampling and appropriate processing, which are both facilitated by ROSE.[34] Immunohistochemistry (IHC) is the most common ancillary test performed on FNA specimens. Most cytopathologists recommend 2 or more dedicated FNA passes to be submitted for IHC testing.[69] IHC is specifically indicated to evaluate tumors of unknown origin and GI subepithelial lesions. For instance, IHC helps distinguish potentially malignant subepithelial tumors, such as GI stromal tumors (GIST), from contamination by GI tract wall muscle cells or benign leiomyomas and schwannomas using stains for anti-CD117, anti-CD34, desmin, muscle-specific actin, and S-100.[31] Other ancillary tests include flow cytometry for evaluating lymphoma, staining or cultures for infectious causes, immunoglobulin G4 staining for autoimmune pancreatitis, and carcinoembryonic antigen analysis of CPTs.[69–71]

Please refer to **Boxes 2** and **3** for a summary of some of the intraprocedural pitfalls that may be encountered.

Box 2
Intraprocedural pitfalls of EUS FNA

Failure to perform comprehensive EUS examination before FNA

- Missing lesions that would indicate a more advanced tumor stage and other preferred site of FNA
- Neglecting to find the most ideal site within the GI tract to access the target lesion

Lesion location contributing to poor echoendoscope position and FNA

- Large luminal diameter and tortuous shape of the stomach and rectum
- Thick gastric wall causing tenting of the needle
- Severe scope angulation (eg, duodenum, fundus) impairing needle advancement
- Overuse of the elevator impairing needle advancement
- Uncinate lesions more challenging to access
- Lesions near the limit of EUS imaging (eg, uncinate, tip of pancreatic tail, right hepatic lobe)

Inability to access the target lesion via the echoendoscope

- Diverticulum (Zenker, duodenal)
- Luminal stricture (benign or malignant)
- Altered anatomy (eg, Roux-en-Y anatomy, gastric bypass, Billroth II, bariatric surgery)
- Retained luminal contents (eg, food, stool) leading to image artifacts or risking adverse events

Inability to access the target lesion via the EUS FNA needle

- Presence of important intervening structures (vessels, ducts, nodes deep to primary tumor, and so forth)
- Lesions located beyond the range of the FNA needle (>7 cm away from the transducer)

Poor EUS imaging of the lesion

- Poor acoustic coupling
- Duodenal diverticulum, small bowel air
- Retained luminal contents that impairs acoustic coupling
- Presence of a stent (eg, bile duct, pancreatic duct, luminal) causing postacoustic shadowing
- Presence of lesion mimicking structures (eg, inflammation, acute or chronic pancreatitis)

Failure to obtain FNAs in an algorithmic manner

- Targeting lesions that would not convey the most advanced tumor stage
- Targeting lesions associated with a lower risk of adverse events

Lesion characteristics that contribute to a difficult FNA

- Smaller lesions that are harder to target
- Larger lesions that contain significant areas of necrosis
- Desmoplastic, indurated lesions that contain more nontumoral supportive tissues (eg, collagen)
- Desmoplastic, indurated lesions that are more difficult to penetrate with the FNA needle
- Desmoplastic, indurated lesions that often produce scant cytologic specimen
- Well differentiated tumors with minimal cellular atypia that require more passes for diagnosis

- Vascular lesions producing a bloody specimen obscuring malignant cells
- Cystic lesions with denuded epithelium that contain scant number of epithelial cells

Improper FNA technique

- Smaller-gauge needles potentially providing inadequate samples
- Larger-gauge needles that are more rigid, particularly difficult to use in transduodenal FNA
- Using a stylet, which may increase the specimen blood content
- Continued use, or too much, of suction that obtains bloody specimens
- Not using, or inadequate, suction when initially obtain scant, dry specimens
- Insufficient techniques (fanning and so forth) to adequately sample the lesion
- Failure to perform quick, jabbing needle movements when necessary
- Too slow a needle movement that may preferentially result in a bloody or inadequate specimen
- Obtaining an inadequate number of needle passes

Incorrect specimen handling and preparation

- Inaccurate labeling of the FNA site and organ or structure being biopsied
- Disproportionate distribution of the specimen onto slides and liquid-based cytology containers
- Delay in distributing the specimen with blood clotting
- Thick, heavy, uneven smearing onto slides
- Drying before fixation
- Improper pattern and timing of staining
- Not providing dedicated passes for cell block and ancillary analyses when necessary

Poor endosonographer and cytopathologist communication

- Failure to communicate the procedure indication
- Not providing information regarding prior therapies (chemotherapy, radiation)
- Not conveying the relative difficulty and risk of FNAs for a particular patient and site
- Failure to alert the cytopathologist when changing the FNA site
- Not providing information on the site of the GI tract the FNA needle traverses

Incorrect or misleading on-site cytopathology review

- Inaccurate interpretation of specimen adequacy by on-site cytotechnologist
- Inaccurate interpretation of malignancy by on-site cytotechnologist
- Telecytology unavailable to assist on-site cytotechnologist review

False-positive and false-negative cytologic results

- Sampling error by the endosonographer
- Cytopathology misinterpretation

Failure to use ancillary techniques

- Not recognizing the utility of ancillary techniques to provide enough samples for pathology review
- Misinterpreting a nonspecific background stain as a positive immunostain

---

Box 3
Cytopathologic interpretive pitfalls by site of EUS FNA

Mediastinum

- Dust-laden macrophages mimicking metastatic melanoma
- Distinguishing mesothelioma cells as a contaminant from malignant mesothelioma

Esophagus

- Benign ulceration with squamous metaplasia mimicking squamous cell carcinoma
- Reactive epithelia mimicking squamous cell carcinoma
- False-positive cytology when traversing Barrett esophagus

Hepatobiliary

- Cholangitis with bile duct stent creating epithelial cells with reactive changes mimicking malignancy
- Difficulty distinguishing poorly differentiated cancers of the hepatobiliary system

Pancreas

- Presence of acute or CP impairing cytologic interpretation
- Sparse specimens from denuded CPT containing little to no epithelium
- Translocation of gut wall epithelium mimicking mucinous cystic tumors
- Pancreatic neuroendocrine tumor misinterpreted as pancreatic splenosis, intrapancreatic lymph nodes, chronic pancreatitis, acinar cell tumors

Subepithelial lesions

- Misinterpretation of muscle cells obtained from the gut wall rather than a subepithelial lesion
- Inability to assess mitotic index (malignant potential) of GISTs using cytology
- Difficulty distinguishing mucosa-associated lymphoid tissue (MALT) lymphoma from chronic gastritis and polymorphous lymphoid appearance
- Frequent need for histology and flow cytometry rather than cytology for MALT lymphoma
- Misinterpreting a gastric pancreatic rest as a pancreatic adenocarcinoma

Lymph nodes

- Malignant lymphoma may require more than cytology alone
- Difficulty distinguishing low-grade follicular lymphoma from reactive lymphadenopathy
- Contamination with dysplastic cells in the presence of a luminal cancer causing false-positive results
- Contamination of benign mucosal glandular cells misinterpreted as malignancy
- Germinal centers mimicking malignancy
- Previously treated lymph nodes with chemoradiation that may give an appearance of epithelial changes with mucinous changes, mimicking cystic pancreatic tumors

---

POSTPROCEDURAL PITFALLS
Suboptimal Timing for Conveying the Results of EUS FNA

There seems to be disparate views in terms of the appropriateness and timing for conveying the results of EUS FNA. Two studies surveyed patients undergoing EUS

FNA of solid pancreatic masses to determine the most appropriate time to discuss the cytopathology results.[72,73] Ninety-two percent of patients in one study had not met the endosonographer before the procedure, and only 28% were aware of the possibility of pancreatic cancer.[73] Despite only meeting the endosonographer briefly, 68% of patients preferred to receive the EUS FNA results immediately from the endosonographer rather than receive later notification from their referring physician with whom they had established a patient-physician relationship. In another study, 71% of patients who were informed of the preliminary FNA results by the endosonographer could remember the correct diagnosis 1 day later, and 84% could recall the diagnosis 1 week after the procedure.[72] Therefore, some think that the endosonographer should discuss the preliminary FNA results with patients immediately after the effects of the sedation have worn off rather than waiting for the referring physician to convey the results. Although this is a reasonable approach, in the authors' practice, they prefer to convey the FNA cytology results only when the cytology review is complete because of the risk of providing incorrect or incomplete information. This approach works well in the authors' practice given that they formally discuss this issue to help set patients' expectations before the procedure. The authors think the delay of 1 to 2 hours that is required until receipt of the final interpretation outweighs the potential harm that occurs when conveying a false-positive or false-negative preliminary reading.

Poor Understanding of Staging Criteria of Malignancy

Because EUS FNA is most commonly performed for GI or thoracic malignancies and often serves as an adjunct to radiologic imaging for staging, it is important for the endosonographer and the multidisciplinary team to understand the TNM staging of these cancers to guide appropriate patient management. Lymph node metastases are particularly important factors contributing to the prognosis and treatment of patients. For example, lymph nodes located in the mesorectum or extending to the internal iliac area in rectal cancer has a better prognosis than lymph node involvement beyond the internal iliac.[74] Without the understanding that lymph node metastases beyond the internal iliac area most likely represent metastatic disease in patients with rectal cancer, these patients may undergo inappropriate surveillance during neoadjuvant therapy or surgical resection.

Poor Understanding of Cytologic Interpretation

Cytologic interpretations are reported as an inadequate sample or negative, atypical, suspicious, or positive for malignancy. In the appropriate clinical setting, specimens reported as negative or positive for malignancy are presumed to be true. Differences in opinion predominately occur in the interpretation of cytology reported as atypical or suspicious for malignancy. Some people would classify atypical as a negative or inadequate sample and suspicious as a positive result, whereas others would interpret both as either a negative or positive result. This difference highlights the importance of providing adequate specimens for the cytopathologist to review to decrease the risk of an atypical or suspicious interpretation. In the authors' practice, unless the clinical history is consistent with malignancy in patients with an EUS FNA resulting in suspicious cytology, they encourage a rebiopsy of any lesion with an inadequate, atypical, or suspicious interpretation.

Please refer to **Box 4** for a summary of some of the postprocedural pitfalls that may be encountered.

Box 4
Postprocedural pitfalls of EUS FNA

Suboptimal timing for conveying the EUS FNA results

- Disparate views on the appropriateness and timing of conveying EUS FNA results for the endosonographer versus referring physician (ie, timeliness vs risk of conveying false information)

Poor understanding of staging criteria

- Misinterpreting the staging criteria and impact on management (eg, external iliac or common iliac vs perirectal lymph nodes)

Poor understanding of cytologic interpretations

- Contrasting view as how best to deal with nonpositive cytologic result (eg, atypical or suspicious)

SUMMARY

EUS FNA is a generally safe and effective modality for tissue acquisition in the diagnosis of GI and some non-GI pathology. However, it is important to remember that pitfalls may be encountered during any aspect of this procedure. Understanding the limitations of EUS FNA allows proper patient education, enhances the diagnostic yield, and may improve safety.

REFERENCES

1. Vilmann P, Jacobsen GK, Henriksen FW, et al. Endoscopic ultrasonography with guided fine needle aspiration biopsy in pancreatic disease. Gastrointest Endosc 1992;38:172–3.
2. Wiersema MJ, Hawes RH, Tao LC, et al. Endoscopic ultrasonography as an adjunct to fine needle aspiration cytology of the upper and lower gastrointestinal tract. Gastrointest Endosc 1992;38:35–9.
3. Lachter J, Rosenthal Y, Kluger Y. A multidisciplinary survey on controversies in the use of EUS-guided FNA: assessing perspectives of surgeons, oncologists and gastroenterologists. BMC Gastroenterol 2011;11:117.
4. Harewood GC, Wiersema LM, Halling AC, et al. Influence of EUS training and pathology interpretation on accuracy of EUS-guided fine needle aspiration of pancreatic masses. Gastrointest Endosc 2002;55:669–73.
5. Eisen GM, Dominitz JA, Faigel DO, et al. Guidelines for credentialing and granting privileges for endoscopic ultrasound. Gastrointest Endosc 2001;54:811–4.
6. Mertz H, Gautam S. The learning curve for EUS-guided FNA of pancreatic cancer. Gastrointest Endosc 2004;59:33–7.
7. Eloubeidi MA, Tamhane A. EUS-guided FNA of solid pancreatic masses: a learning curve with 300 consecutive procedures. Gastrointest Endosc 2005;61:700–8.
8. Wilson JA, Hoffman B, Hawes RH, et al. EUS in patients with surgically altered upper GI anatomy. Gastrointest Endosc 2010;72:947–53.
9. Lee JH, Topazian M. Pancreatic endosonography after Billroth II gastrectomy. Endoscopy 2004;36:972–5.
10. Gleeson FC, Kipp BR, Caudill JL, et al. False positive endoscopic ultrasound fine needle aspiration cytology: incidence and risk factors. Gut 2010;59:586–93.

11. Gimeno-Garcia AZ, Elwassief A. How to improve the success of endoscopic ultrasound guided fine needle aspiration cytology in the diagnosis of pancreatic lesions. J Interv Gastroenterol 2012;2:31–6.
12. Chang KJ. Maximizing the yield of EUS-guided fine-needle aspiration. Gastrointest Endosc 2002;56:S28–34.
13. Prasad P, Schmulewitz N, Patel A, et al. Detection of occult liver metastases during EUS for staging of malignancies. Gastrointest Endosc 2004;59:49–53.
14. Polkowski M, Larghi A, Weynand B, et al. Learning, techniques, and complications of endoscopic ultrasound (EUS)-guided sampling in gastroenterology: European Society of Gastrointest Endosc (ESGE) technical guideline. Endoscopy 2012;44:190–206.
15. Agarwal B, Gogia S, Eloubeidi MA, et al. Malignant mediastinal lymphadenopathy detected by staging EUS in patients with pancreaticobiliary cancer. Gastrointest Endosc 2005;61:849–53.
16. Hahn M, Faigel DO. Frequency of mediastinal lymph node metastases in patients undergoing EUS evaluation of pancreaticobiliary masses. Gastrointest Endosc 2001;54:331–5.
17. Faigel DO, Ginsberg GG, Bentz JS, et al. Endoscopic ultrasound-guided real-time fine-needle aspiration biopsy of the pancreas in cancer patients with pancreatic lesions. J Clin Oncol 1997;15:1439–43.
18. Wiersema MJ, Vilmann P, Giovannini M, et al. Endosonography-guided fine-needle aspiration biopsy: diagnostic accuracy and complication assessment. Gastroenterology 1997;112:1087–95.
19. Afify AM, al-Khafaji BM, Kim B, et al. Endoscopic ultrasound-guided fine needle aspiration of the pancreas. Diagnostic utility and accuracy. Acta Cytol 2003;47:341–8.
20. Ramesh J, Varadarajulu S. How can we get the best results with endoscopic ultrasound-guided fine needle aspiration? Clin Endosc 2012;45:132–7.
21. Levy MJ, Wiersema MJ. EUS-guided Trucut biopsy. Gastrointest Endosc 2005;62:417–26.
22. Siddiqui AA, Brown LJ, Hong SK, et al. Relationship of pancreatic mass size and diagnostic yield of endoscopic ultrasound-guided fine needle aspiration. Dig Dis Sci 2011;56:3370–5.
23. Tournoy KG, Ryck FD, Vanwalleghem L, et al. The yield of endoscopic ultrasound in lung cancer staging: does lymph node size matter? J Thorac Oncol 2008;3:245–9.
24. Uehara H, Ikezawa K, Kawada N, et al. Diagnostic accuracy of endoscopic ultrasound-guided fine needle aspiration for suspected pancreatic malignancy in relation to the size of lesions. J Gastroenterol Hepatol 2011;26:1256–61.
25. Haba S, Yamao K, Bhatia V, et al. Diagnostic ability and factors affecting accuracy of endoscopic ultrasound-guided fine needle aspiration for pancreatic solid lesions: Japanese large single center experience. J Gastroenterol 2013;48(8):973–81.
26. Rong L, Kida M, Yamauchi H, et al. Factors affecting the diagnostic accuracy of endoscopic ultrasonography-guided fine-needle aspiration (EUS-FNA) for upper gastrointestinal submucosal or extraluminal solid mass lesions. Dig Endosc 2012;24:358–63.
27. Wee E, Lakhtakia S, Gupta R, et al. Endoscopic ultrasound guided fine-needle aspiration of lymph nodes and solid masses: factors influencing the cellularity and adequacy of the aspirate. J Clin Gastroenterol 2012;46:487–93.

28. Weynand B, Deprez P. Endoscopic ultrasound guided fine needle aspiration in biliary and pancreatic diseases: pitfalls and performances. Acta Gastroenterol Belg 2004;67:294–300.

29. Binmoeller KF, Rathod VD. Difficult pancreatic mass FNA: tips for success. Gastrointest Endosc 2002;56:S86–91.

30. Orell SR. Pitfalls in fine needle aspiration cytology. Cytopathology 2003;14: 173–82.

31. Jenssen C, Dietrich CF. Endoscopic ultrasound-guided fine-needle aspiration biopsy and trucut biopsy in gastroenterology-an overview. Best practice & research. Clin Gastroenterol 2009;23:743–59.

32. Schmidt RL, Witt BL, Matynia AP, et al. Rapid on-site evaluation increases endoscopic ultrasound-guided fine-needle aspiration adequacy for pancreatic lesions. Dig Dis Sci 2013;58:872–82.

33. Petrone MC, Arcidiacono PG, Carrara S, et al. Does cytotechnician training influence the accuracy of EUS-guided fine-needle aspiration of pancreatic masses? Dig Liver Dis 2012;44:311–4.

34. da Cunha Santos G, Ko HM, Saieg MA, et al. "The petals and thorns" of ROSE (rapid on-site evaluation). Cancer Cytopathol 2013;121:4–8.

35. Olson MT, Ali SZ. Cytotechnologist on-site evaluation of pancreas fine needle aspiration adequacy: comparison with cytopathologists and correlation with the final interpretation. Acta Cytol 2012;56:340–6.

36. Puli SR, Bechtold ML, Buxbaum JL, et al. How good is endoscopic ultrasound-guided fine-needle aspiration in diagnosing the correct etiology for a solid pancreatic mass?: a meta-analysis and systematic review. Pancreas 2013;42:20–6.

37. Puli SR, Batapati Krishna Reddy J, Bechtold ML, et al. Endoscopic ultrasound: it's accuracy in evaluating mediastinal lymphadenopathy? A meta-analysis and systematic review. World J Gastroenterol 2008;14:3028–37.

38. Thornton GD, McPhail MJ, Nayagam S, et al. Endoscopic ultrasound guided fine needle aspiration for the diagnosis of pancreatic cystic neoplasms: a meta-analysis. Pancreatology 2013;13:48–57.

39. Dumonceau JM, Koessler T, van Hooft JE, et al. Endoscopic ultrasonography-guided fine needle aspiration: relatively low sensitivity in the endosonographer population. World J Gastroenterol 2012;18:2357–63.

40. Eloubeidi MA, Jhala D, Chhieng DC, et al. Yield of endoscopic ultrasound-guided fine-needle aspiration biopsy in patients with suspected pancreatic carcinoma. Cancer 2003;99:285–92.

41. Kliment M, Urban O, Cegan M, et al. Endoscopic ultrasound-guided fine needle aspiration of pancreatic masses: the utility and impact on management of patients. Scand J Gastroenterol 2010;45:1372–9.

42. Woolf KM, Liang H, Sletten ZJ, et al. False-negative rate of endoscopic ultrasound-guided fine-needle aspiration for pancreatic solid and cystic lesions with matched surgical resections as the gold standard: one institution's experience. Cancer Cytopathol 2013;121(8):449–58.

43. Recine M, Kaw M, Evans DB, et al. Fine-needle aspiration cytology of mucinous tumors of the pancreas. Cancer 2004;102:92–9.

44. Eloubeidi MA, Wallace MB, Reed CE, et al. The utility of EUS and EUS-guided fine needle aspiration in detecting celiac lymph node metastasis in patients with esophageal cancer: a single-center experience. Gastrointest Endosc 2001;54:714–9.

45. Korenblit J, Anantharaman A, Loren DE, et al. The role of endoscopic ultrasound-guided fine needle aspiration (EUS-FNA) for the diagnosis of intra-abdominal lymphadenopathy of unknown origin. J Interv Gastroenterol 2012;2:172–6.

46. Byrne MF, Gerke H, Mitchell RM, et al. Yield of endoscopic ultrasound-guided fine-needle aspiration of bile duct lesions. Endoscopy 2004;36:715–9.

47. DeWitt J, Misra VL, Leblanc JK, et al. EUS-guided FNA of proximal biliary strictures after negative ERCP brush cytology results. Gastrointest Endosc 2006;64:325–33.

48. Ohshima Y, Yasuda I, Kawakami H, et al. EUS-FNA for suspected malignant biliary strictures after negative endoscopic transpapillary brush cytology and forceps biopsy. J Gastroenterol 2011;46:921–8.

49. Khashab MA, Kim K, Lennon AM, et al. Should we do EUS/FNA on patients with pancreatic cysts? The incremental diagnostic yield of EUS over CT/MRI for prediction of cystic neoplasms. Pancreas 2013;42:717–21.

50. Levy MJ, Gleeson FC, Campion MB, et al. Prospective cytological assessment of gastrointestinal luminal fluid acquired during EUS: a potential source of false-positive FNA and needle tract seeding. Am J Gastroenterol 2010;105:1311–8.

51. Vander Noot MR 3rd, Eloubeidi MA, Chen VK, et al. Diagnosis of gastrointestinal tract lesions by endoscopic ultrasound-guided fine-needle aspiration biopsy. Cancer 2004;102:157–63.

52. Fritscher-Ravens A, Brand L, Knofel WT, et al. Comparison of endoscopic ultrasound-guided fine needle aspiration for focal pancreatic lesions in patients with normal parenchyma and chronic pancreatitis. Am J Gastroenterol 2002;97:2768–75.

53. Varadarajulu S, Tamhane A, Eloubeidi MA. Yield of EUS-guided FNA of pancreatic masses in the presence or the absence of chronic pancreatitis. Gastrointest Endosc 2005;62:728–36 [quiz: 751, 753].

54. Jhala NC, Jhala DN, Chhieng DC, et al. Endoscopic ultrasound-guided fine-needle aspiration. A cytopathologist's perspective. Am J Clin Pathol 2003;120:351–67.

55. Lim LG, Lakhtakia S, Ang TL, et al. Factors determining diagnostic yield of endoscopic ultrasound guided fine-needle aspiration for pancreatic cystic lesions: a multicentre Asian study. Dig Dis Sci 2013;58(6):1751–7.

56. Dumonceau JM, Polkowski M, Larghi A, et al. Indications, results, and clinical impact of endoscopic ultrasound (EUS)-guided sampling in gastroenterology: European Society of Gastrointestinal Endoscopy (ESGE) clinical guideline. Endoscopy 2011;43:897–912.

57. Rogart JN, Loren DE, Singu BS, et al. Cyst wall puncture and aspiration during EUS-guided fine needle aspiration may increase the diagnostic yield of mucinous cysts of the pancreas. J Clin Gastroenterol 2011;45:164–9.

58. Hong SK, Loren DE, Rogart JN, et al. Targeted cyst wall puncture and aspiration during EUS-FNA increases the diagnostic yield of premalignant and malignant pancreatic cysts. Gastrointest Endosc 2012;75:775–82.

59. Atiq M, Bhutani MS, Bektas M, et al. EUS-FNA for pancreatic neuroendocrine tumors: a tertiary cancer center experience. Dig Dis Sci 2012;57:791–800.

60. Ardengh JC, de Paulo GA, Ferrari AP. EUS-guided FNA in the diagnosis of pancreatic neuroendocrine tumors before surgery. Gastrointest Endosc 2004;60:378–84.

61. Gines A, Vazquez-Sequeiros E, Soria MT, et al. Usefulness of EUS-guided fine needle aspiration (EUS-FNA) in the diagnosis of functioning neuroendocrine tumors. Gastrointest Endosc 2002;56:291–6.

62. Stelow EB, Bardales RH, Stanley MW. Pitfalls in endoscopic ultrasound-guided fine-needle aspiration and how to avoid them. Adv Anat Pathol 2005;12:62–73.

63. Tatsas AD, Owens CL, Siddiqui MT, et al. Fine-needle aspiration of intrapancreatic accessory spleen: cytomorphologic features and differential diagnosis. Cancer Cytopathol 2012;120:261–8.

64. Ardengh JC, Lopes CV, Kemp R, et al. Pancreatic splenosis mimicking neuroendocrine tumors: microhistological diagnosis by endoscopic ultrasound guided fine needle aspiration. Arq Gastroenterol 2013;50:10–4.

65. Rodriguez E, Netto G, Li QK. Intrapancreatic accessory spleen: a case report and review of literature. Diagn Cytopathol 2013;41:466–9.

66. Frankel WL. Update on pancreatic endocrine tumors. Arch Pathol Lab Med 2006;130:963–6.

67. Labate AM, Klimstra DL, Zakowski MF. Comparative cytologic features of pancreatic acinar cell carcinoma and islet cell tumor. Diagn Cytopathol 1997; 16:112–6.

68. Stelow EB, Bardales RH, Shami VM, et al. Cytology of pancreatic acinar cell carcinoma. Diagn Cytopathol 2006;34:367–72.

69. Kulesza P, Eltoum IA. Endoscopic ultrasound-guided fine-needle aspiration: sampling, pitfalls, and quality management. Clin Gastroenterol Hepatol 2007; 5:1248–54.

70. Yasuda I, Goto N, Tsurumi H, et al. Endoscopic ultrasound-guided fine needle aspiration biopsy for diagnosis of lymphoproliferative disorders: feasibility of immunohistological, flow cytometric, and cytogenetic assessments. Am J Gastroenterol 2012;107:397–404.

71. Sodikoff JB, Johnson HL, Lewis MM, et al. Increased diagnostic yield of endoscopic ultrasound-guided fine needle aspirates with flow cytometry and immunohistochemistry. Diagn Cytopathol 2012. [Epub ahead of print].

72. Early DS, Janec E, Azar R, et al. Patient preference and recall of results of EUS-guided FNA. Gastrointest Endosc 2006;64:735–9.

73. Siddiqui UD, Rossi F, Padda MS, et al. Patient preferences after endoscopic ultrasound with fine needle aspiration (EUS-FNA) diagnosis of pancreas cancer: rapid communication valued over long-term relationships. Pancreas 2011;40: 680–1.

74. Akiyoshi T, Watanabe T, Miyata S, et al. Results of a Japanese nationwide multi-institutional study on lateral pelvic lymph node metastasis in low rectal cancer: is it regional or distant disease? Ann Surg 2012;255:1129–34.

Future Directions in EUS-guided Tissue Acquisition

Pierre H. Deprez, MD, PhD

KEYWORDS

- Endoscopic ultrasound • Fine-needle aspiration • Molecular testing • Elastography

KEY POINTS

- EUS-FNA tissue acquisition will still be the gold standard in the future.
- All other promising techniques, such as optical biopsies with nCLE, contrast-enhanced EUS, and elastography, will enable the clinician to focus on specific areas and targets for FNA rather than replace tissue acquisition.
- Even more material will be needed for immunochemistry and molecular testing to improve malignancy diagnosis and guide targeted therapy.
- Therefore, new needles are needed with an improved design, mainly to increase the amount of material sampled in fewer passes with optimal safety for the patient.

INTRODUCTION

Endoscopic ultrasound (EUS) has revolutionized the ability to diagnose and stage cancers of the gastrointestinal tract and assess the pancreas. EUS fine-needle aspiration (FNA) is now routinely used to acquire tissue from different tissue structures located in the vicinity of the gastrointestinal tract. The pancreas and lymph nodes are the most common organs targeted in EUS-FNA with excellent sensitivity and specificity.[1] For the diagnosis of solid pancreatic masses a recent medical literature review showed a 78% to 95% sensitivity, 75% to 100% specificity, and 78% to 95% accuracy confirming that EUS-FNA is an effective and safe method to obtain a cytologic diagnosis of pancreatic tumors.[2] EUS-FNA has also been proved to increase the accuracy of lymph node staging and thereby reduce the number of unnecessary surgical interventions. A meta-analysis from 76 studies on mediastinal lymph nodes demonstrated that FNA improved the sensitivity from 84% to 88% and specificity from 88% to 96% compared with EUS imaging alone.[3]

Nevertheless, the negative predictive value of EUS-FNA is low, especially for the diagnosis of pancreatic neoplasms. The same is true for other targets, such as lung cancer during endoscopic bronchial US. Pathologists are well aware of the limited

Disclosure: The author disclosed no financial relationships relevant to this publication.
Department of Hepato-gastroenterology, Cliniques Universitaires Saint-Luc, Université Catholique de Louvain, Avenue Hippocrate 10, Brussels 1200, Belgium
E-mail address: pdeprez@uclouvain.be

Gastrointest Endoscopy Clin N Am 24 (2014) 143–149
http://dx.doi.org/10.1016/j.giec.2013.08.004   giendo.theclinics.com

amount of tumor that may actually be present in diagnostic samples used for lung cancer diagnosis. A recent study demonstrated that the median percentage of tumor present in malignant samples was little more than 20% when squamous cell or adeno-carcinoma was diagnosed, whereas this figure was only 10% in non–small cell lung cancer cases.[4]

The emergence of selective, targeted therapies, directed toward a particular molec-ular characteristic of an individual patient's tumor, is now driving the need for biomarker identification and testing in several cancer types. This means that the tech-nique needs improvement to provide more material, in fewer passes, with more flexible, sharp, and clearly echovisible needles and with a similar safety. Future needs and expectancies are as follows:

- Either acquisition of more material
  - To allow for cytology, histology, immunocytochemistry or histochemistry, and molecular biology
  - With fewer passes
  - With needles that are flexible, sharp, echovisible, and cost effective
  - With auxiliary devices inserted in the needle (brush, forceps, and so forth)
- Or avoidance of tissue acquisition or limited tissue acquisition with the help of ancillary techniques, such as
  - Optical biopsies
  - Contrast-enhanced US
  - Elastography
  - Other tissue analysis techniques.

These issues may be combined or selectively used for specific lesions. Future trends include the following:

- Improvement of the sampling technique
- Development of new needles
- Widespread use of liquid phase cytology and cell blocks
- Combination of cytology and histology with FNA biopsy
- Use of immunocytochemistry and histochemistry
- Use of polymerase chain reaction, flow cytometry
- Use and validation of molecular markers
- More routine use of ancillary techniques, such as elastography, contrast-enhanced EUS
- Optical biopsies obtained through the needle

IMPROVEMENT OF SAMPLING AND SAMPLE PROCESSING

Previous papers in this issue address the key points to improve tissue acquisition. The first step is appropriate training. The American Society for Gastrointestinal Endos-copy recommends a minimum of 150 supervised cases, of which 75 should be pancreaticobiliary, and 50 EUS-FNA should be performed.[5] The next step is a puncture technique adapted to the target: choice of needle caliber; with or without suction depending on tissue hardness and vascularization; number of passes (presence of a cytopathologist in the room or not); and most importantly use of the fanning technique (at individual passes, the needle should be positioned at different areas within the mass and then moved back and forth two to three times in each area to procure tissue).[6] The technique may also be adapted to the needle used, histology needles needing less suction and passes through the targeted tissue.[7]

Getting a sample in the appropriate target is only the first step. Next steps depend on the quality and amount of the material and on its adequate processing. A case is made in many expert centers for a more widespread use of immunocytochemistry/histochemistry, even in cases where the pathologist is more confident of the diagnosis on morphologic grounds. Indeed, a lower threshold for the use of immunochemistry may be appropriate and improve diagnostic accuracy.[4] The use of immunochemistry to augment morphologic diagnosis on small tissue samples consumes much more tissue than conventional morphologic diagnosis alone. The routine preparation of cell blocks from fluid and needle aspiration cytology samples will also assist in providing extra-diagnostic material for other tests. The importance of tissue preparation and preservation is emphasized by the emergence of predictive molecular marker testing.[8,9]

NEED FOR NEW NEEDLES

During the past two decades, EUS-FNA has evolved to become a major tool for tissue acquisition. However, clinicians have been working with the same needles with known limitations: 25-G and 22-G procure small amounts of material with little information on tissue architecture, and 19-G needles are difficult to use for transduodenal access because of the inherent rigidity induced by large caliber and the torqued echoendoscope.

To overcome this technical challenge, a new 19-G fine-needle biopsy device (Pro-Core; Cook Endoscopy, Winston-Salem, NC) was recently developed with reverse bevel technology to enable the acquisition of core specimens for histologic analysis. In a large prospective study from Europe, histologic samples were obtained successfully with the fine-needle biopsy needle in most patients, with diagnostic accuracy of more than 90%.[10] However, technical difficulties were still encountered in the performance of transduodenal passes. A more flexible 19-G needle (Flex 19; Boston Scientific, Natick, MA) made of nitinol was recently tested in difficult-to-access lesions. A preliminary onsite cytologic diagnosis was established in 92% of patients and a histologic diagnosis in 95%. A definitive diagnosis was achieved in 100% of cases when both cytology and histology were combined. The authors encountered no technical difficulty or needle dysfunction in any procedures.[11]

Other manufacturers are also developing new needles: needles with side ports (Olympus, Tokyo, Japan); and multiple low cost needles that can be rapidly exchanged through the single delivery system, reducing the down time between needle passes, which improves the clinical workflow (Beacon Endoscopic, Newton, MA).

There is room for improvement: intermediate-size needles (20-G or 21-G) might be more useful for combined cytology and histology sampling, or use of auxiliary devices inside the sheath of the 19-G needle.[12,13] Perhaps in a more futuristic vision we should abandon our bulky scopes and move to more flexible luminal robotic-driven devices to access and puncture potential targets.

OPTICAL BIOPSY RATHER THAN TISSUE ACQUISITION?

Confocal laser endomicroscopy (CLE) is a novel endoscopic method that allows intravital microscopy of the human gastrointestinal mucosa during ongoing endoscopy, enabling real-time optical biopsy.[14] Recent technology allows a confocal miniprobe (pCLE) to be passed through the biopsy channel of the endoscope, whereas the optical biopsy images are usually coregistered with the histopathology results performed at the conclusion of pCLE imaging.[15,16] Based on the same CLE system, microprobe-based CLE has been combined with EUS-guided puncture of pancreatic cystic lesions, a procedure termed needle-based CLE (nCLE). It provides real-time microscopic imaging of pancreatic cysts during EUS-FNA procedures and it is compatible with 19-G needles. Although follow-up trials are to be awaited, nCLE may prove valuable not only in the evaluation of cystic lesions, but also focal masses.[17,18]

WHAT ABOUT MOLECULAR TESTING?

These technical novelties place the endosonographer at a crossroad: should we abandon tissue acquisition or will we need more material for molecular testing, flow cytometry, polymerase chain reaction, and other new techniques? Pancreatic cancer is a good example in gastroenterology to illustrate this point. It is characterized by a variety of molecular alterations, and therefore, identification and quantification of potential molecular markers for pancreatic cancer on cellular samples obtained by EUS-FNA could be a promising approach for the diagnosis of malignancy.[19,20] EUS-FNA allows the extraction of sufficient quantities of RNA to perform quantitative real-time polymerase chain reaction analysis, low-density array, and other molecular testing techniques. Broad panel microsatellite loss and *k-ras* point mutation analysis can be reliably performed on EUS-FNA samples from pancreatic masses and improves the diagnostic accuracy.[21] Another approach is to use mismatch excision repair, a DNA repair system that eliminates mismatched base pairs and plays an important role in maintaining genomic integrity. The use of mismatch excision repair genes for the differentiation between pseudotumoral chronic pancreatitis and pancreatic cancer using a minimally invasive sampling technique could be a promising technique.[8] Large-scale gene analysis may therefore become a powerful method for diagnosis of malignancy, to predict prognosis, invasion, and metastasis through the identification of biomarkers.

Is there enough tumor tissue on which to perform these tests? There is no definitive answer to this question; how much is enough? RNA and DNA may be extracted from a sample containing few tumor cells, but will be contaminated by nucleic acids from normal cells. How do we interpret the test result, especially if the molecular marker is not unique to the malignant process? Few studies reporting biomarker data address these questions; some barely mention test methodology. In the same way, studies have shown that there is no tumor present in a significant proportion of EUS-FNA samples, highlighting the risk of submitting such tissue samples for molecular diagnosis without prior pathologic examination to confirm the presence of tumor.[4]

EUS ELASTOGRAPHY: GOOD EXAMPLE OF A FACILITATING ANCILLARY TECHNIQUE

EUS-FNA may provide false-negative results for malignancy, may be unfeasible because of technical problems or interposed malignant tissue and vascular structures, and is associated with a small but not insignificant morbidity. As a result of efforts to overcome these limitations, most recent US image processors provide elastography, a technique that allows the imaging and quantifying of the hardness of lesions with dedicated software.[22] The principle of EUS elastography is based on the assumption that compression of a target tissue by an echoendoscopic probe produces a smaller strain (ie, displacement of one tissue structure by another) in hard tissue than in soft tissue. Thus, by calculating the elasticity of tissue, it is possible to differentiate benign (soft) tissue from malignant (hard) tissue.[23] The recent introduction of second-generation EUS elastography allows quantitative analysis of tissue stiffness; the simplest of these methods uses the ratio of the elasticity of a given mass to that of a selected reference region within adjacent soft tissue, the so-called strain ratio. The most significant advantage of EUS elastography is that it can be performed in real time during a diagnostic examination with immediate information provided to the endosonographer.

Several reports showed a high sensitivity and specificity of EUS elastography in differentiating between benign and malignant solid pancreatic masses. All of these studies underscored the capability of elastography to help the endosonographer to select a site where FNA can be performed with improved diagnostic yield, particularly in patients with either necrotic tumors or possible cancer in a background of diffuse inflammatory change.[24,25]

Some studies, however, did not confirm the high specificity and accuracy shown by expert centers. In the largest single-center study to date, the diagnostic utility of quantitative EUS elastography for discriminating pancreatic masses was modest, suggesting that it may only supplement rather than supplant the role of pancreatic tissue sampling in the future.[26,27] The true value of the technique in patients in whom FNA failed to provide a diagnosis or in those with underlying chronic pancreatitis has not been consistently proved. EUS elastography will therefore never replace tissue acquisition but should be part of the endosonographer's armamentarium to improve its diagnostic performance.[28] It may indeed help to detect and delineate pancreatic tumors and improve FNA targeting, at a low cost and without the need for extensive training in the use of the software, which will be available on most processors.[29]

SUMMARY

Will EUS-FNA tissue acquisition still be the gold standard in the next future? The answer is, yes, mainly because of the development of molecular testing. All other promising techniques, such as optical biopsies with nCLE, contrast-enhanced EUS, and elastography, will enable the clinician to focus on specific areas and targets for FNA rather than replace tissue acquisition. Therefore, there is still a need for new needles with an improved design, mainly to increase the amount of material sampled in fewer passes with optimal safety for the patient.

REFERENCES

1. Wiersema MJ, Hawes RH, Tao LC, et al. Endoscopic ultrasonography as an adjunct to fine needle aspiration cytology of the upper and lower gastrointestinal tract. Gastrointest Endosc 1992;38:35–9.
2. Hewitt MJ, McPhail MJ, Possamai L, et al. EUS-guided FNA for diagnosis of solid pancreatic neoplasms: a meta-analysis. Gastrointest Endosc 2012;75:319–31.
3. Puli SR, Batapati Krishna Reddy J, Bechtold ML, et al. Endoscopic ultrasound: it's accuracy in evaluating mediastinal lymphadenopathy? A meta-analysis and systematic review. World J Gastroenterol 2008;14:3028–37.
4. Kerr KM. Personalized medicine for lung cancer: new challenges for pathology. Histopathology 2012;60:531–46.
5. Eisen GM, Dominitz JA, Faigel DO, et al. American Society for Gastrointestinal Endoscopy. Guidelines for credentialing and granting privileges for endoscopic ultrasound. Gastrointest Endosc 2001;54:811–4.
6. Bang JY, Magee SH, Ramesh J, et al. Randomized trial comparing fanning with standard technique for endoscopic ultrasound-guided fine-needle aspiration of solid pancreatic mass lesions. Endoscopy 2013;45:445–50.
7. Polkowski M, Larghi A, Weynand B, et al. Learning, techniques, and complications of EUS-guided sampling endoscopic ultrasound (EUS)-guided sampling in gastroenterology: European Society of Gastrointestinal Endoscopy (ESGE) Technical Guideline. Endoscopy 2012;44:190–205.

8. Gheonea DI, Ciurea ME, Săftoiu A, et al. Quantitative RT-PCR analysis of MMR genes on EUS-guided FNA samples from focal pancreatic lesions. Hepatogastroenterology 2012;59:916–20.

9. Costache MI, Iordache S, Karstensen JG, et al. Endoscopic ultrasound-guided fine needle aspiration: from the past to the future. Endosc Ultrasound 2013; 2(2):77–85.

10. Iglesias-Garcia J, Poley JW, Larghi A, et al. Feasibility and yield of a new EUS histology needle: results from a multicenter, pooled, cohort study. Gastrointest Endosc 2011;73:1189–96.

11. Varadarajulu S, Bang JY, Hebert-Magee S. Assessment of the technical performance of the flexible 19-gauge EUS-FNA needle. Gastrointest Endosc 2012; 76(2):336–43.

12. Bruno M, Bosco M, Carucci P, et al. Preliminary experience with a new cytology brush in EUS-guided FNA. Gastrointest Endosc 2009;70:1220–4.

13. Aparicio JR, Martínez J, Niveiro M, et al. Direct intracystic biopsy and pancreatic cystoscopy through a 19-gauge needle EUS (with videos). Gastrointest Endosc 2010;72:1285–8.

14. Kiesslich R, Burg J, Vieth M, et al. Confocal laser endoscopy for diagnosing intraepithelial neoplasias and colorectal cancer in vivo. Gastroenterology 2004;127: 706–13.

15. ASGE Technology Committee, Kantsevoy SV, Adler DG, Conway JD, et al. Confocal laser endomicroscopy. Gastrointest Endosc 2009;70:197–200.

16. Kiesslich R, Neurath MF. Endomicroscopy is born: do we still need the pathologist? Gastrointest Endosc 2007;66:150–3.

17. Konda VJ, Aslanian HR, Wallace MB, et al. First assessment of needle-based confocal laser endomicroscopy during EUS-FNA procedures of the pancreas (with videos). Gastrointest Endosc 2011;74:1049–60.

18. Saftoiu A, Vilmann P, Bhutani MS. Endoscopic ultrasound-guided confocal laser endomicroscopy: using the optical needle into the acoustic haystack. Eur J Ultrasound 2012;33:607–10.

19. Laurell H, Bouisson M, Berthelemy P, et al. Identification of biomarkers of human pancreatic adenocarcinomas by expression profiling and validation with gene expression analysis in endoscopic ultrasound-guided fine needle aspiration samples. World J Gastroenterol 2006;12:3344–51.

20. Bournet B, Pointreau A, Souque A, et al. Gene expression signature of advanced pancreatic ductal adenocarcinoma using low density array on endoscopic ultrasound-guided fine needle aspiration samples. Pancreatology 2012;12:27–34.

21. Ogura T, Yamao K, Sawaki A, et al. Clinical impact of K-ras mutation analysis in EUS-guided FNA specimens from pancreatic masses. Gastrointest Endosc 2012;75:769–74.

22. Ophir J, Céspedes I, Ponnekanti H, et al. Elastography: a quantitative method for imaging the elasticity of biological tissues. Ultrason Imaging 1991;13:111–34.

23. Săftoiu A, Vilmann P, Gorunescu F, et al. European EUS Elastography Multicentric Study Group. Accuracy of endoscopic ultrasound elastography used for differential diagnosis of focal pancreatic masses: a multicenter study. Endoscopy 2011; 43:596–603.

24. Mei M, Ni J, Liu D, et al. EUS elastography for diagnosis of solid pancreatic masses: a meta-analysis. Gastrointest Endosc 2013;77:578–89.

25. Iglesias-Garcia J, Larino-Noia J, Abdulkader I, et al. Quantitative endoscopic ultrasound elastography: an accurate method for the differentiation of solid pancreatic masses. Gastroenterology 2010;139:1172–80.

26. Janssen J, Schlörer E, Greiner L. EUS elastography of the pancreas: feasibility and pattern description of the normal pancreas, chronic pancreatitis, and focal pancreatic lesions. Gastrointest Endosc 2007;65:971–8.
27. Dawwas MF, Taha H, Leeds JS, et al. Diagnostic accuracy of quantitative EUS elastography for discriminating malignant from benign solid pancreatic masses: a prospective, single-center study. Gastrointest Endosc 2012;76:953–61.
28. Hirche TO, Ignee A, Barreiros AP, et al. Indications and limitations of endoscopic ultrasound elastography for evaluation of focal pancreatic lesions. Endoscopy 2008;40:910–7.
29. Deprez PH. EUS elastography: is it replacing or supplementing tissue acquisition? Gastrointest Endosc 2013;77:590–2.

Index

Note: Page numbers of article titles are in **boldface** type.

A

Adenocarcinoma
  bile duct
    evaluation of
      in assessment of diagnostic sufficiency and options for handling EUS-FNA
        specimen, 54
  ductal
    evaluation of
      in assessment of diagnostic sufficiency and options for handling EUS-FNA
        specimen, 50
Adequacy assessment
  of diagnostic sufficiency and options for handling EUS-FNA specimen, 37–38
Appropriate fixation
  in handling of cytology sample, 21
Aspirate(s)
  semisolid
    in assessment of diagnostic sufficiency and options for handling EUS-FNA
      specimen, 39

B

B-cell lymphoma
  non-Hodgkin
    evaluation of
      in assessment of diagnostic sufficiency and options for handling EUS-FNA
        specimen, 47
Bile duct
  acute inflammation of
    evaluation of
      in assessment of diagnostic sufficiency and options for handling EUS-FNA
        specimen, 47
Bile duct adenocarcinoma
  evaluation of
    in assessment of diagnostic sufficiency and options for handling EUS-FNA
      specimen, 54
Biliary tumors
  upper
    staging of, 12
Biopsy(ies)
  EUS-FNA
    techniques for, **83–107**. *See also* Endoscopic ultrasound–guided fine-needle biopsy
      (EUS-FNB), techniques for

Gastrointest Endoscopy Clin N Am 24 (2014) 151–160
http://dx.doi.org/10.1016/S1052-5157(13)00122-0
1052-5157/14/$ – see front matter © 2014 Elsevier Inc. All rights reserved.

giendo.theclinics.com

Moving?

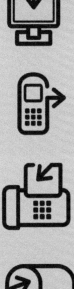

Printed and bound by CPI Group (UK) Ltd, Croydon, CR0 4YY

03/10/2024

01040493-0014